WHAT DOCTORS FEEL

Also by Danielle Ofri

Singular Intimacies: Becoming a Doctor at Bellevue

*Incidental Findings: Lessons from My Patients
in the Art of Medicine*

Medicine in Translation: Journeys with My Patients

WHAT DOCTORS FEEL

How Emotions Affect the Practice of Medicine

Danielle Ofri, MD

BEACON PRESS
BOSTON

Beacon Press
Boston, Massachusetts
www.beacon.org

Beacon Press books
are published under the auspices of
the Unitarian Universalist Association of Congregations.

26 25 24 23   12 11 10 9

This book is printed on acid-free paper that meets the uncoated paper
ANSI/NISO specifications for permanence as revised in 1992.

To protect privacy, all patients' names have been changed (with the
exception of Julia Amparo-Alvarado and Isaac Edwards, whose names and
stories are already in the public record from news media). Additionally,
other identifying characteristics have been changed. Real names are used for
doctors who gave permission. For those doctors who preferred anonymity,
only first names (pseudonyms) are used.

Text design and composition by Kim Arney

Parts of chapter 5 were published as Danielle Ofri,
"Ashamed to Admit It: Owning Up to Medical Error,"
Health Affairs 29 (2010): 1549–51.

John Stone, "Gaudeamus Igitur," *Journal of the American Medical Association*
249, no. 13 (1983): 1741–42. Copyright © 1983 American Medical
Association. All rights reserved. Reprinted with permission.

Library of Congress Cataloging-in-Publication Data
Ofri, Danielle.
What doctors feel : how emotions affect the practice of medicine / Danielle Ofri.
p. ; cm.
Includes bibliographical references.
ISBN 978-0-8070-3330-2 (paperback : alk. paper)
I. Title.   1. Attitude of Health Personnel—Personal Narratives.   2. Physicians—
psychology—Personal Narratives.   3. Emotions—Personal Narratives.
4. Empathy—Personal Narratives.   5. Interprofessional Relations—Personal
Narratives.   6. Physician-Patient Relations—Personal Narratives.
610.69'5—dc23   2012049349

For Naava, Noah, and Ariel

Contents

Introduction
Why Doctors Act That Way   1

Chapter 1
The Doctor Can't See You Now   6

   Julia, part one   23

Chapter 2
Can We Build a Better Doctor?   29

   Julia, part two   60

Chapter 3
Scared Witless   64

   Julia, part three   95

Chapter 4
A Daily Dose of Death   98

   Julia, part four   122

Chapter 5
Burning with Shame   124

   Julia, part five   140

Chapter 6
Drowning   143

 Julia, part six   170

Chapter 7
Under the Microscope   173

 Julia, part seven   202

Afterword   210

Acknowledgments   213

Notes   215

Index   221

Why Doctors Act That Way

The experiences of medical training and the hospital world have been extensively documented in books, television, and film. Some of this has been probing and incisive, and some has been entertaining nonsense. Much has been written about what doctors do and how they frame their thoughts. But the emotional side of medicine—the parts that are less rational, less amenable to systematic intervention—has not been examined as thoroughly, yet it may be at least as important.

The public remains both fascinated and anxious about the medical world—a world with which everyone must eventually interact. Within this fascination is a frustration that the health-care system does not function as ideally as people would like. Despite societal pressures, legislative reforms, and legal wrangling, doctors don't always live up to these ideals. I hope to delve beneath the cerebral side of medicine to see what actually makes MDs tick.

One might reasonably say, *I don't give a damn how my doctor feels as long as she gets me better.* In straightforward medical cases, this line of thinking is probably valid. Doctors who are angry, nervous, jealous, burned out, terrified, or ashamed can usually still treat bronchitis or ankle sprains competently.

The problems arise when clinical situations are convoluted, unyielding, or overlaid with unexpected complications, medical errors, or psychological components. This is where factors other than clinical competency come into play.

At this juncture in our society's history, nearly every patient—at least those in the developed world—can have access to the same fund of medical knowledge that doctors work from. Anyone can search WebMD for basic information or PubMed for the latest research. Medical textbooks and journals are available online. The relevant issue—the one that has the practical impact on the patient—is how doctors *use* that knowledge.

There has been a steady stream of research into how doctors think. In his insightful and practically titled book *How Doctors Think,* Jerome Groopman explored the various styles and strategies that doctors use to guide diagnosis and treatment, pointing out the flaws and strengths along the way. He studied the cognitive processes that doctors use and observed that emotions can strongly influence these thought patterns, sometimes in ways that gravely damage our patients. "Most [medical] errors are mistakes in thinking," Groopman writes. "And part of what causes these cognitive errors is our inner feelings, feelings we do not readily admit to and often don't even recognize."[1]

Research bears this out.[2] Positive emotions tend to be associated with a more global view of a situation ("the forest") and more flexibility in problem solving. Negative emotions tend to diminish the importance of the bigger picture in favor of the smaller details ("the trees"). In cognitive psychology studies, subjects with negative emotions are more prone to anchoring bias—that is, latching on to a single detail at the expense of others. Anchoring bias is a potent source of diagnostic error, causing doctors to stick with an initial impression and avoid considering conflicting data. Subjects with positive emotions are also prone to bias; they are more likely to succumb to attribution bias. In medicine, this is the tendency to attribute a disease to who the patient is (a drug user, say) rather than what the situation is (exposure to bacteria, for example).

This is not to say that positive emotions are better or worse than negative emotions—both are part of the normal human spectrum. But if you consider the range of cognitive territory that doctors traverse with their patients—genetic testing, ordinary screenings, invasive procedures, ICU monitoring, and end-of-life decisions—you can appreciate how the final outcomes can be strongly influenced by a doctor's emotional state.

Neuroscientist Antonio Damasio describes emotions as the "continuous musical line of our minds, the unstoppable humming."[3] This basso continuo thrums along while doctors make a steady stream of conscious medical decisions. How this underlying bass line affects our actions as doctors—and the net effect on our patients (and on doctors when we ourselves become patients!)—is what intrigues me.

By now, even the most hard-core, old-school doctors recognize that emotions are present in medicine at every level, but typically this is lumped in with the catch-all of stress or fatigue, with the unspoken assumption that with enough self-discipline, physicians can corral and master these irritants.

The emotional layers in medicine, however, are far more nuanced and pervasive than we may like to believe. In fact, they can often be the dominant players in medical decision-making, handily overshadowing evidenced-based medicine, clinical algorithms, quality-control measures, even medical experience. And this can occur without anyone's conscious awareness.

It could easily be argued that doctors are no more emotionally complex than accountants, plumbers, or the cable-repair guy, but the net result of doctors' behavior—logical, emotional, irrational, or otherwise—can have life-and-death consequences for patients, which is to say, for all of us.

We all want excellent medical care for ourselves and our families, and we'd like to assume that the best care comes from the doctors with the best training, or the most experience, or the best *U.S. News & World Report* rating. However, the myriad effects of emotional underpinnings can confound all of these factors.

Despite this, the conventional stereotype that doctors are fairly emotionless continues to maintain its hold. Many trace this back to the eminent Canadian physician Sir William Osler, often considered the father of modern medicine for such revolutionary ideas as whisking medical students out of the staid classroom and bringing them to the bedside to learn medicine by examining actual patients. The current educational system of clinical clerkships and residency training is largely attributed to Osler, as are hundreds of snappy quotations. His continuing influence is apparent in the scores of diseases, endless libraries, and numerous medical buildings, hospital wings, societies, and awards that bear his name.

On May 1, 1889, Dr. Osler stood before the graduating medical class at the University of Pennsylvania and delivered a valedictory— and now canonical—speech entitled "Aequanimitas."[4] He stressed to these fledgling doctors that "a certain measure of insensibility is not only an advantage, but a positive necessity in the exercise of a calm judgment."

While Osler may not have created these attitudes, he neatly encapsulated the general feeling about how doctors should behave. Though he did warn against "hardening the human heart," the stereotype of the detached, coolheaded physician springs from this idea of equanimity.

Popular culture has embodied this. Television doctors from Ben Casey to Gregory House are detached from their patients, lauded for their technological and diagnostic acumen. Even the selflessly idealist doctors (in *Arrowsmith*, *Middlemarch*, and *Cutting for Stone*) and the bitingly sarcastic doctors (in *M*A*S*H*, *House of God*, and *Scrubs*) maintain an equanimitous distance from their patients.

Every hospital dutifully includes the word *compassion* somewhere in its mission statement. Every medical school rhapsodizes about the ideals of caring. But the often unspoken (and sometimes spoken) message in the real-life trenches of medical training is that doctors shouldn't get too emotionally involved with their patients. Emotions cloud judgment, students are told. Any component of a curriculum upon which interns slap the "touchy-feely" label is doomed in terms of attendance. Hyperefficient, technically savvy medical care is still prized over all else.

But no matter how it's portrayed, and no matter how many high-tech tools enter the picture, the doctor-patient interaction is still primarily a human one. And when humans connect, emotions by necessity weave an underlying network. The most distant, aloof doctor is subject to the same flood of emotions as the most touchy-feely one. Emotions are in the air just as oxygen is. But how we doctors choose—or choose not—to notice and process these emotions varies greatly. And it is the patient at the other end of the relationship who is affected most by this variability.

This book is intended to shed light on the vast emotional vocabulary of medicine and how it affects the practice of medicine at all levels. Hopefully, the next time we find ourselves in a patient gown, we'll better understand the workings of those who care for us. "Cognition and emotion are inseparable," Groopman observes. "The two mix in every encounter with every patient."[5] In some scenarios, this mix is highly beneficial to patients. In others, it can be calamitous.

Understanding the positive and negative influence of emotions in the doctor-patient interaction is a crucial element in maximizing the quality of medical care. Every patient deserves the best possible care that doctors can offer. Learning to recognize and navigate the emotional subtexts is a critical tool on both sides of the exam table.

CHAPTER I

The Doctor Can't
See You Now

Which one would she be? I hovered by the door to the emergency room, my eyes darting from one patient to the next. As a first-year medical student whose entire medical career thus far had existed inside cavernous, windowless lecture halls, the chaos of the ER and my role here terrified me. I gazed at a shivering Hispanic teenager in jeans and a sweatshirt filling out forms with a nurse: Was it her? I saw a college-age Asian woman in a heavy overcoat following an orderly to radiology: Was it her? There was a lumpy form curled up on a stretcher in the far corner. Perhaps that was her. Would it show?

Three months before, I'd signed up to be a volunteer rape-crisis counselor at Bellevue Hospital. Along with a half a dozen other medical students and a sprinkling of hospital employees, I'd sat through a six-week training program on how to support a victim of sexual assault through the difficult ER experience, how to act as an advocate—sometimes as a buffer—during the interactions with doctors, nurses, police, family.

Each morning, the beeper was passed from one volunteer to the next. "Did you get called?" we asked each other anxiously. The very act of carrying a beeper, of being potentially responsible for something, made us all nervously excited.

At 3:00 a.m., a beeper went off for the first time ever in my life, a searing jumble of excitement and terror. I frantically pulled on clothes and then sprinted over to the hospital in the darkness. And now, standing by the door, peering in at this bizarre hive of activity,

I fought to settle my jangling nerves. How would I find her? What would I say to her? What exactly qualified me to be in this role?

I took a deep breath, then stepped tentatively into the swirl of bodies and business, heading toward the triage desk. I found the charge nurse and explained why I was there. She grabbed a clipboard and scanned the names, pressing the eraser end of a pencil to the corner of her lip. "Josephine Hamlin, that's yours," she said finally, inclining the pencil toward a disheveled black woman a few feet away. "GYN's already been here. Just needs to get cleaned up."

The woman was clearly homeless, with shaggy, matted hair and dirt-encrusted clothing of indeterminate color. She sat hunched on the edge of the stretcher, her gaunt legs drooping toward the floor, feet stuffed into unlaced construction boots without socks. The weather-beaten cragginess of her face obscured her age. Desolate eyes stared vacantly into space. Her body appeared frozen in mid-breath; whether inhalation or exhalation, it was impossible to tell.

Gingerly, I took several steps toward her. As I drew closer, a pungent odor enveloped me, the fetid smell of an unwashed body and moldering clothes. I pressed forward, despite the nausea that was gathering at the back of my throat. Then a faint movement near her shoulder caught my eye, and I stiffened in my spot as a roach emerged from a fold in her threadbare sweater. It paused, as though taking in the scene, then sauntered placidly down her arm. It hesitated midway, and then finally rounded her elbow and disappeared into a layer of clothing.

I stood frozen, my stomach clenched to keep its contents in place. My eyes raced from corner to corner of the ER, searching for someone or something to tell me what to do. I tried to step forward, but my legs wouldn't budge. The grimy smell seemed to intensify, surging in brackish waves that threatened to drown me.

I knew that I had to swallow it all back, that I had to continue my approach toward this woman. This is what I'd signed on for when I enrolled in medical school—to help patients in need, no matter who they were or what they looked like. The Hippocratic oath, the oath of Maimonides—this was what these professional oaths were written for.

Yet my body refused to move. The revolting smell, capped by the appearance of a genuine New York City roach, was simply too much for me. I could tell from the unaltered blankness of her stare that I hadn't yet registered on her horizon, that I was still part of the blur and buzz of the emergency room . . . that there was still time to hide.

I groped behind me and inched backward until I reached the triage desk and could squeeze my inadequacy safely behind the Formica counter. I sank into a 1950s-era office chair and covered my mouth with my hands, unsure if I could keep from vomiting.

Panicky thoughts jittered through my mind. What I was going to do? This was my patient, after all. This was a human being who had just been violated in the most horrible manner. It was my job to go there and help her. This was what it meant to be a doctor.

Yet all I could do was cringe behind the desk, gutlessly pretending to examine paperwork. It's not that I was obsessive about cleanliness or needed everything to be pristine. By this point in my academic career, I'd dissected pigs, frogs, sheep brains, cow eyeballs. Even prior to medical school, I'd dissected plenty of human cadavers, having been an undergraduate teaching assistant in both anatomy and neuroanatomy. I was completely at ease with bisected pelvises and cross-sectioned livers. During my PhD research in neuroscience, I pulverized cow brains from the local kosher butcher and beheaded live mice by the dozen. Squeamish I was not.

But the rancid smell of this patient undid me. And cockroaches had somehow never been subsumed into my childhood passion for all things animal. The combination thereof activated a primal revulsion that I simply could not quiet with my rational thoughts.

Three minutes later, a nurse's aide—an older Haitian woman—approached the patient. The aide reached out and took the patient's hand in hers. She spoke softly and I watched as she coaxed the patient's gaze up to hers. The aide reached out her other hand and gently smoothed the patient's stiff, tangled hair.

Slowly the patient stood, listing slightly to the left. The aide stepped in closer, supporting the woman as they began walking toward the shower room, their heads nearly touching. As they passed the triage desk, I could hear the aide's encouraging voice: "You'll feel so much better after a shower. And we can get you some fresh clothes." The aide's arm was secure around the patient's shoulders. "I know a quiet place where you can rest afterward. Don't worry; I'll stay with you."

I sat hidden behind the desk, awed and humbled. As their distance from me grew and the potent stench concomitantly receded, I could finally exhale. I sank back in my chair, realizing how much I needed to learn about medicine.

—⁂—

When I look back at my medical training from my current vantage point—nearly three decades from that moment in the ER—I can pinpoint seminal moments of clinical development: the first time jumbled susurrations in the earpieces of my stethoscope organized themselves into an identifiable cardiac murmur, the first time a glistening newborn was guided into my gloved and apprehensive hands, the first time a needle guided by my fingers punctured a human being's skin.

Each of these moments represented another rung on the steep ladder of medical training and was, in fact, transforming. After each hurdle, I was not the same person as before; I was one step closer to becoming that still murky image of a doctor, and one step farther removed from the unformed student who had entered medical school. These epochal experiences were so momentous that I can still remember the details of the place where each one occurred, and, more important, I remember each teacher who guided me through.

That moment in the ER with the nurse's aide was another of those formative events of doctorhood. I was experiencing a most visceral lesson in empathy. That aide's act of compassion left me breathless. I knew that she was smelling the same stink I smelled, seeing the same grime and wretchedness. Yet she went to the woman without any evident hesitation. She not only stepped forward but also gave of herself to the patient. In that moment, she personified for me what it meant to be a caregiver.

To have compassion—literally, as its Latin roots suggest, to be able to suffer with—one must have empathy. It is impossible to fake compassion; empathy is a necessary prerequisite.

Empathy is one of those odd concepts that is so central to human interaction, so obviously a requirement in medicine, something we intuitively know when we see, yet so difficult for many to precisely define. For now I'll sidestep the detailed philosophical discussion about whether empathy is an emotion or a cognition and stick with how most people define it: the ability to see and feel from another person's perspective.

Specifically for medicine, empathy is about recognizing and appreciating a patient's suffering. The oath of Maimonides, which many graduating classes recite upon receiving their medical degrees, sums it up succinctly: "May I never see in the patient anything but a fellow creature in pain." Empathy requires being attuned to the patient's perspective and understanding how the illness is woven into this particular person's life. Last—and this is where doctors often stumble—empathy requires being able to communicate all of this to the patient.

Doctors tend to find empathy easiest when patients' suffering seems to make sense—pain from a broken leg, for example—or when patients seem deserving, victims of bad luck rather than their own egregious behavior.

It's far more challenging when the suffering doesn't make sense to the doctor, when there isn't an obvious wound, or a tumor on the X-ray, or a lab value that objectively indicates disease. Doctors fall short on empathy when pain seems out of proportion to the illness, when the patient appears to have an ulterior motive, or when the disease is self-inflicted, from "slothful" or "reckless" habits.

There can be a gut reaction toward patients who are smelly, or dirty, or nauseating, as I experienced in the ER. Like all human beings, doctors can be repulsed by people and things that are disgusting. But physically repulsive conditions are an occupational hazard of medicine, and doctors are supposed to be able to control their reactions. The first time I opened a dressing to see a throng of maggots gamboling within a skin ulcer, I thought I'd be the next admission to the hospital. But by the end of internship, I was flushing out maggots with brisk squirts of saline, even appreciating that their snacking on the necrotic tissue had lightened my workload of cleaning the wound.

Most doctors manage to acclimatize to the gorier aspects of medicine, but it can take a prodigious effort to overcome reactions to the nonmedical things we find repellent. Some people—like the nurse's aide that day in the ER—can do it effortlessly, but for others, it takes prodding and self-discipline.

My team once admitted a patient with skin ulcers—a condition whose anodyne name belies the range of possible severity. Skin ulcers are incredibly common, but it was the specifics of how the resident reported the case to me that seared it in my memory. "His ulcers look incompatible with life," she said without a trace of irony in her tone. "I don't understand how he's still alive."

Incompatible with life? Those words chilled me.

When I went to see the patient, I understood immediately why she'd chosen that phrasing. James Easton was a frail, elderly man from a nursing home. *Skin-and-bones* would have been a lavish description. Mr. Easton's face was deflated of muscle tone, hollowed of expression, parched of animus. What few fibrils of muscle he possessed hung limply off his skeleton. But it was the skin ulcers that were beyond anything I'd ever seen.

Ulcers coursed down his thighs and calves, filleting them open into canyons of decay. The walls of the crevices dug deep into the tissue, eviscerating everything in their path. The femur and tibia bones were visible to the naked eye. Even parts of the pelvic bones were exposed. It was like a surrealist's take on an anatomy lesson.

My mouth hung open; I was unable to fathom what combination of disease, neglect, microbes, genetics, and bad luck had brought him to this state. His physical condition and his severe dementia made him nearly incapable of communication. Whether he understood any of what transpired around him was impossible to determine. How he was still alive was incomprehensible to me; there was so little left of him. There was no person inside to talk to, barely any physical body to examine. He hardly seemed human.

The ulcers were indeed incompatible with life, and if left alone, they would snuff out what scant life force remained. Antibiotics and wound care—the usual treatment for infected ulcers—were ineffective at this advanced stage. The only recourse was amputation. But because the ulcers ran all the way to the tops of his legs, the legs had to actually be disarticulated right from the hip joint.

If it were possible, Mr. Easton looked even less human after the amputations—a torso with two spindly arms, not even stumps for legs. If the first step of empathy is identifying with a patient, of trying to imagine yourself in that person's shoes, our empathy skills were sorely tested.

—◊◊◊—

Beyond physical aspects of a patient that can stymie doctors' empathy, there are also personality characteristics to which doctors react with less empathy than they should—patients who are hostile or manipulative, patients who are painfully shy and reveal nothing of themselves, patients who seem entitled and arrogant. Right after residency, I took a summer job in a family practice in Long Island, covering Friday and Saturday office hours for a physician I'll call Dr. Palmer. I was in a middle-class town that in summers swelled to twice its size with wealthy Manhattanites whose beach houses lined the crystalline shores.

Needless to say, the setting was quite different from my training at Bellevue. It wasn't just a matter of switching from an uninsured, largely immigrant population to an affluent, stable population, most of whom spoke English. It was a veritable culture shock—medically—to go from a world of critically ill hospitalized patients to a calm outpatient suburban setting of basically healthy people. My final month in residency had been spent in the ICU dealing with septic shock, severe hemorrhages, and multisystem organ failure. Now my patients came for a miscellanea of sore throats, rashes, and sprained ankles—ailments too pedestrian to even make it onto the medical radar during residency. But I quickly became a master at tick removal and identification of Lyme disease.

One day, a healthy-looking woman in her early forties came for an appointment. Cynthia Landon asked me to prescribe fen-phen (fenfluramine-phentermine), a weight-loss pill that was being heavily marketed at the time.

The whole idea of weight-loss pills had always rubbed me the wrong way; it seemed like a Band-Aid approach to a problem that usually resulted from a lifetime of eating patterns and inactivity, so already my hackles were up. From my vantage point across the desk, I thought she certainly seemed to be within a normal weight range. "Why do you want to take weight-loss pills?" I asked her, somewhat incredulously.

She grasped a handful of her stomach and said ruefully, "I've been trying to get rid of these extra pounds after having kids."

I leaned closer to see what she was gripping, and it looked like a regular amount of stomach to me. After three years of round-the-clock AIDS, cancer, congestive heart failure, and cirrhosis, it was hard to get worked up over a couple of middle-aged pounds. I mean, really . . .

"Your weight looks pretty reasonable to me," I said in what I thought was a pleasant, objective voice. It was a compliment, actually, because frankly she looked fine for her age. "Plus these pills don't do much. Whatever pound or two they take off will come right back as soon as you stop. It's not a permanent solution. And every medication has side effects to consider. Have you tried—"

But before I could get to any discussion about diet and exercise, Ms. Landon cut me off. "Dr. Palmer prescribes fen-phen for me," she said curtly. "I need a prescription from you, not a lecture."

I was taken aback by the sharp edge in her voice. I was even more taken aback that Dr. Palmer prescribed those pills for someone who wasn't obese. But I was a temp here. These weren't my patients; they were Dr. Palmer's, and my job was to continue his usual care in his absence. This week he and his family were on vacation, and I was trying my best to act as a worthy substitute. But now I was getting annoyed.

"Every medication is a serious proposition," I said. "You can't just—"

"Dr. Palmer is my doctor," she said angrily. "My insurance covers the medication, and this is what I need."

Suddenly I began to feel unsure of myself. Dr. Palmer had decades of experience with outpatient medicine. All I had was three years in the hospital; what did I know about office-based medicine? Maybe this was what outpatient doctors did? Maybe fen-phen was appropriate for mild middle-age weight gain, and I was just being naïve? And if this was what the patient had been taking, who was I to stop it? Would that be "abandoning" a patient in the midst of her care?

But it didn't sit right with me. So I finally said, "Maybe it's best that you make an appointment with Dr. Palmer to talk about it with him."

"He's away this week," she snapped back at me, "and the secretary told me that he's completely booked the week he comes back."

I could feel the pressure like a barometric surge. This patient clearly wasn't going to back down. Well, damn it, neither was I. *If she thinks she can railroad me just because I'm the new doc in town . . .*

Then I glanced up at the clock and thought about the full waiting room outside. I didn't want to spend all morning fighting this out; there was too much else to do. I could just give her the prescription and be done with it. How much harm could thirty pills do? I probably wasn't ever going to see her again. What would it matter in the long run? But then I would have been manipulated by this patient. That alone was getting me steamed.

"I'm sorry," I finally said, my voice now as curt as hers. "But in my professional opinion, fen-phen would not be medically indicated in this situation."

Ms. Landon glared at me for one long hard moment, then pursed her lips and stood up. She grabbed her handbag and exited the room without a word or glance. I felt shaken, but also proud that I'd resisted her pressure and stood my ground.

Summer was just waning when an article appeared in the *New England Journal of Medicine* showing that fen-phen might cause valvular heart disease. Shortly thereafter, the medication was pulled from the market. I felt vindicated, even smug. *I told you so,* I imagined saying to Ms. Landon.

But as I think about this episode years later, I realize that I let my own anger at being manipulated dominate the interaction. My sense of feeling threatened made it hard to be empathic toward Cynthia Landon. I wasn't able to step past my own issues—both my lack of confidence as a new doctor, and my personal bias against the medication itself—and try to understand her issues. Perhaps she had an eating disorder that had drastically altered her perception of her weight. Perhaps there were other underlying issues at play, emotional issues more complex than a few extra pounds post-kids.

But we never got that far. I wasn't able to be particularly empathic with her not just because I was angry but also because she seemed so entitled. She apparently felt that she could just march right in and demand whatever she wanted. She struck me, at the moment, as spoiled and vain. All I could think of was how many patients at Bellevue were truly sick and really needed medical care. Her selfish use of the medical system for her petty, superficial issues—not to mention the drug companies' exploitation of this—disgusted me.

But maybe none of that was true. Maybe underneath the seemingly superficial concerns were serious issues that were crying out for attention. Maybe I'd just screwed up and missed a biggie. Depression. Suicidality. Domestic violence. Bulimia. Drug addiction. Alcoholism. Any of these serious (and potentially fatal) conditions could have been lurking beneath a simple request for diet pills. Even wealthy, insured people with extravagant beach homes get sick. Even annoying, selfish, and entitled people need care. But my empathy was stymied that day by the emotions that ignited between us, and I wasn't able to explore beneath the surface.

My only consolation was that perhaps I'd spared her from the side effects of fen-phen. A few years later, I learned that I might have even spared her from the side effects of Dr. Palmer. A DWI conviction revealed a serious alcohol problem. Complaints were filed by several patients, and his practice came under investigation. Ultimately, his medical license was suspended because his medical practice "did not meet an acceptable standard of care."

—∽—

In general, empathy is easier the more we can identify with someone. When we can genuinely envision ourselves in a situation, it's possible to intuit what that person's suffering might feel like. When the gap between doctor and patient is larger—for whatever reason—the challenge is thornier.

Doctors tend to come from a narrower spectrum of society than patients. Though medical schools are more diverse than they once were, most doctors still hail from wealthier (and healthier) middle-class backgrounds and have far less experience with illness, disability, economic instability, unemployment, and prejudice than their patients do. Patients can seem so different from doctors that the doctors can have trouble identifying with them.

Some of the challenges to empathy arise from cultural and language barriers. Many Asian patients I've worked with, for example, are very reticent about admitting pain and can keep up a stoic front despite severe illness. Doctors stop "seeing" the pain of these patients and invest their concern in others. At the other end of the emotional spectrum, Hispanic patients have a reputation for being very vocal about their symptoms (whence arises the hospital-slang diagnosis Hispanic Hysterical Syndrome). These patients never seem to stop complaining, and doctors rapidly stop listening.

Both of these scenarios could be written off as stereotypical—and they certainly do not capture the wide range of actual responses—but they do represent examples in which physicians can lose a connection to their patients' suffering because of culturally nuanced differences in manners of expression. I have one patient who has been in my practice for many years. Maríssima Alvarez is a sixty-two-year-old woman from Ecuador who is fortunate enough to be free of the diabetes, hypertension, and heart disease that plague most of my other patients her age. But she does have chronic aches and pains that bring her to my office with an impressive frequency. She probably has some combination of arthritis and a chronic pain syndrome. I respect this and try to take her symptoms seriously—though I find reassurance in the fact that her overall health has remained stable in the decade I've taken care of her. The problem is that every symptom is "the worst ever."

In Spanish, suffixes are added to words to form superlatives, and that is Ms. Alvarez's standard way of speaking. Her stomach pains are not *malo* (bad), they are *malísimo* (the worst). Her headache is never *grande* (big), but *grandote* (huge). The burning in her stomach is not *caliente* (hot), but *calientísima* (the hottest ever). She's never feeling *débil* (weak), but *débilísima* (the weakest ever).

As Ms. Alvarez's doctor, I am supposed to examine every medical complaint with equal concern, because one of them just might represent something serious or life-threatening. But when every symptom ranks 10 (or more) on the scale of 1 to 10, this can be challenging, to say the least.

Whenever I hear her voice on the phone, I can't help the inner groan, the here-we-go-again reaction. I've caught myself starting to tune her out, mumbling or nodding absently to each of her "worst ever" symptoms. (And it hasn't escaped my notice that her first name—Maríssima, which rhymes with her real first name—is prestocked with the superlative suffix -ísima.)

Ms. Alvarez is my personal challenge for empathy. The temptation is to write off most of what she says, and I could argue that there is a medical basis for this: if every organ system were indeed at its worst-ever state—for ten years, no less—she'd be in the ICU or dead. It can be rough going to maintain both composure and empathy in these situations, but a doctor's failure to do that is probably the number one reason why patients feel dissatisfied with their physicians and end up doctor-shopping endlessly.

I know that Ms. Alvarez is trying her best to impress upon me the magnitude of her distress. She is clearly worried that I won't see it if she doesn't paint it vividly enough. Part of me wonders whether it would be helpful to explain to patients like Ms. Alvarez that these efforts can actually work against them, that consistently inflating or exaggerating symptoms can diminish the patient's credibility and erode the physician's empathy. But while the patient does bear some responsibility, I believe that the onus falls more heavily on the doctor to be attuned to the factors—cultural, ethnic, or just personal style— that influence how patients present their symptoms.

—∾—

Ethnic differences are but one example of cultural divides between doctors and patients. Another cultural divide—arguably far vaster— turns up in the context of illnesses that are perceived to be self-induced. Doctors have notorious contempt for alcoholics, drug addicts, and morbidly obese patients, and they often make little effort to conceal it. By unspoken rules, these patients are considered fair game for jokes by medical personnel at all levels. Hospital slang for such patients reflects not just disgust but also anger and resentment. It's not uncommon to hear an obese patient referred to as a beached whale, or a homeless alcoholic called a shpoz or dirtbag.

Physicians are the products of an educational system that demands years of self-discipline and delayed gratification. Despite the knowledge that addiction and obesity have at least some biological components, many doctors still unconsciously—and often consciously—view these conditions as purely a result of sloth, self-indulgence, greed, malingering, and apathy. Respect and appreciation for the ravages of these illnesses—especially when the patients themselves often appear not to—is more than some physicians can muster.

There's no doubt that patients with addictions are probably the most difficult type of patients to work with. Beyond the biologic components of their illnesses, these patients are often saddled with complex overlays of depression, childhood mistreatment, sexual abuse, socioeconomic ills, and personality disorders, not to mention a fragmented medical system with meager options for treating addiction.

Whatever inroads a doctor, therapist, program, or the patient herself might make is handily inundated by the multitude of counterforces that seem to conspire against successful treatment. It's no wonder that doctors-in-training rapidly assume a nihilist attitude toward addicts and invest as little as possible in their care.

The residents and students that we train at Bellevue Hospital see so many alcohol (ETOH, or ethanol) withdrawal patients that these cases cease to have any individuality. If the admitting diagnosis is ETOH WD, the team typically takes a cursory history and then just dials up the benzodiazepines until the shakes subside. The days are counted until the patient can walk steadily and thus be discharged. Attempts at drug-rehabilitation referrals are halfhearted at best. Empathy is in short supply.

It's not hard to see why otherwise conscientious and empathic young doctors behave this way. The ETOH-WD patients are typically surly, smelly, and demanding. Nearly all of them march right out of the hospital to their next drink and then get readmitted two weeks later. Many of these patients sport records of multi-city tours of rehabs, all of which seem to have amounted to nothing. Quite a few are skilled manipulators for oxycodone and Valium. Many have managed to obtain public assistance or disability but appear to do nothing but drink or take drugs. It is easy for doctors—who usually approach life with a pull-yourself-up-by-your-own-bootstraps attitude—to become resentful and disgusted by these seemingly parasitic, self-serving moochers.

John Carello was one such patient I took care of several years ago. The resident on my team announced our new admission by drily stating that this was Mr. Carello's fifty-seventh admission to Bellevue Hospital. Every admission was for either overdose or withdrawal from opiates—heroin or oxycodone. Today was an overdose, and the official treatment plan consisted of letting Mr. Carello sleep it off. I scanned the voluminous chart; it looked as though each resident had simply copied the medical history from the prior admission, and it was hard to blame them because nothing really changed from one admission to the next.

For teaching rounds each day, the team would pick one or two of our new admissions for us to review in depth, and usually they selected the most unusual case, the most interesting case, or the sickest patient. As a challenge that day, I suggested that we discuss Mr. Carello for rounds—arguably the most boring admission on the service. I was also challenging myself, as the attending, to find teaching points in even the most ordinary of cases.

I took the team to the bedside, wondering if I was making an enormous mistake that I would later regret. I had an image of a grouchy patient rambling on about nothing, unwilling or unable to answer any questions accurately. I could envisage the team shuffling their feet, grimacing at the putrid odor, surreptitiously glancing at their to-do lists, wishing they'd brought coffee, counting down the minutes until I released them from this torture, thinking up ever more scathing comments to write in their end-of-rotation evaluations of me.

Mr. Carello, a forty-nine-year-old white man, appeared exactly as billed—disheveled, unshaven, glassy-eyed, with the characteristic beaten-down-by-life look. His skin had the pallid, pasty look of worn-out china. I tried to gather as many chairs as possible so that we wouldn't be hovering over him, but there were only a handful. The medical students were stuck squashed against the back wall.

The interview did not start out promisingly. Most of my questions were met with one-word answers or grunts. Mr. Carello could cite the standard data—stints at rehab, assorted methadone regimens, prison terms—but the facts blended into a bleak, familiar tableau. Though I kept my gaze directed at Mr. Carello (who in turn stared mainly at the ceiling), I could sense a restlessness around me as my team began to lose focus. I was neither connecting with the patient nor educating my trainees. It was just the morass of addiction—never-ending for the patient, never-ending for the medical team. Though I kept up the earnest questions and the concerned tone of voice, nihilism steadily crept up on me.

Then a question came to me, one I'd never thought of before. "Mr. Carello," I said, "I know you have been using drugs for many years. But might you be able to tell us the precise moment when you knew that you were addicted?"

Mr. Carello hoisted himself up onto his elbows and looked at me as though he'd only now noticed someone at his bedside. He squinted, extending the shadow of his brow farther down along his ashy cheeks. From his angled perch he cast a sweeping glance at the semicircle of white-coated doctors around his bed. The shuffling halted.

"When I got addicted?" he asked, focusing again on me, his jaw starting to move left and right like he was weighing the question.

"Yes," I said, surprised that this line of questioning was somehow making me feel uncomfortable. "Mostly we doctors only see patients when they are already well into their illness. We also see patients at checkups when they are perfectly healthy. But we are never present at the exact transition point. Could you take us there, to the exact moment when you knew you were addicted?"

I wasn't sure if this was an unfair question, given his years of addiction, the scores of dramas large and small, the muddles of drug-addled memories, the blackouts beyond recall, but I let the question hang in the air while he pondered, masticating in silence.

He hitched himself up a few degrees more, clamped his lips, then released them. His jaw was less fidgety once he started to speak. "Oh yes," he said, "there was an exact moment." His voice narrowed, gaining more focus as he spoke. "It was early April—I know because those trees that are everywhere in the city had their white blossoms. Looks like snow on the trees for about two weeks, until all the leaves come out and then they're just ordinary trees.

"Anyway, it was early April, and I was driving north on the Henry Hudson Parkway in this old Nissan I'd bought from a construction buddy. I was driving up toward Yonkers, to a barbecue my brother was hosting for his kid's birthday. The trees were full of snow on both sides of the parkway. Like the Christmas display at Macy's." He paused for a second, perhaps savoring the recollection, perhaps straightening out his chronology.

"Then all of a sudden, I needed a hit. It came on a like a tidal wave, but I needed it and I needed it now. But more importantly, I *wanted* it. I wanted it more than anything. I wanted it more than seeing my brother, more than seeing my little nephew. At that moment, it was the only thing in the world for me." Mr. Carello paused, and his jaw resumed its jerky, side-to-side swing. I wondered if it was a muscular tic, maybe a side effect of his drugs or one of the many psych meds he'd received over the years.

"I remember turning that Nissan around," he continued, "looping around on West 158th Street. As soon as I had that car heading southbound, I knew I was addicted. It was like some magnet pulling me back to that shithole downtown where my dealer was. But I had to get there. And that's how I knew. Simple as that."

He stilled his restless jaw with effort. "It was like God reached a hand down and flicked a finger at my car, at my life—flicked me in the other direction, and then there was no going back. The Big Guy just spun me downtown, and I've been heading that way ever since."

The room was pin-drop silent after that. The interns and students seemed frozen in place. I, too, was riveted by the specificity of the memory, of the tangible scene he created. I imagined that each of us in the room was envisioning what it would be like to sit in that car and feel mysterious and inexorable forces turning it around, to feel entirely powerless to control events.

After our interview, we filed out of Mr. Carello's room and regrouped at the end of the hallway. The change in the team was palpable. For the first time, we had some insight—even if slight—into what Mr. Carello's life was like. It was the genesis of true empathy. To be given the chance to slip into his shoes made us view our patient differently. After that, there was no further eye-rolling or offhand disparaging comments when we discussed his case. Team members stopped in his room more frequently to chat, and he in turn was far more cooperative and pleasant. This nascent empathy surely wouldn't eradicate the years of addiction overnight, but it's hard to imagine that his illness would have a chance of remitting without it.

Julia, part one

I remember the precise day that Julia Amparo-Alvarado fell off the Starling curve. It was a Monday morning, one of those crisp fall days in which even New York City seems to brim with autumnal exuberance. The garden in front of Bellevue was lush with gold and scarlet. A gentle soughing of boughs beguiled the senses to ignore the gritty First Avenue traffic just beyond the wrought-iron fence. An illusion of New England tranquillity was granted by the cidery pungence of turning leaves.

A stream of doctors, nurses, technicians, patients, administrators, and orderlies was pouring into the hospital to start the day, but a handful of us had been lured by the spell of the garden, an incongruously sylvan opal set in the concrete skeleton of Manhattan.

Thus, my excuse for being late to the always-scintillating Monday-morning staff meeting was purely horticultural, or so I told myself as I dashed though the clinic waiting room toward the conference room. I skidded to a halt, though, when I spied Julia sitting by herself in the empty waiting room. Her petite body was sunk low in the chair, and her breaths had an odd thickness about them, a deliberateness I had not seen before. Her skin seemed sallower, bereft of animus. Julia had been my patient for close to a decade, and the Starling curve had been instrumental in keeping her alive for all these years—along with her medications, her cardiologists, and her sheer tenacity.

The Starling curve is a tenet of cardiac physiology familiar to all medical students. When the heart is stretched by increased blood volume entering the ventricles, it contracts more forcefully in order to maintain that all-important equilibrium of blood coming into the heart and blood going out.

Julia's heart had been weakening over the years due to lousy genetic luck. For inexplicable reasons, the muscle fibers of Julia's heart had begun to flag when she was in her early thirties, leading to fluid overload in her lungs and lower legs—congestive heart failure (CHF). But because her body was otherwise healthy, it pulled all its physiologic aces out of its sleeve, corralling all possible compensatory mechanisms to keep blood flowing to the vital organs: The heart stepped up its pace to fire out the blood more quickly. Her body's network of veins clenched up to encourage blood return to the heart. The heart fibers thickened—much like a flexed biceps— to push more blood out. The left ventricle of the heart morphed its shape to become more spherical and less cylindrical, thus reducing stress on its walls.

But Julia's disease was relentless, and the muscle fibers of her heart gradually faltered, stretching and thinning out her overtaxed left ventricle. The Starling curve was her last remaining physiologic ace. Much like a stretched-out rubber band that will spring back with increased force, her stretched-out muscle fibers actually worked harder to squeeze more. The nature of the Starling curve is that the farther the cardiac fibers are stretched, the harder the heart can squeeze.

But this ace—and, indeed, all her physiologic aces—was tailored by evolution to deal with *acute* heart failure, things like infections, mammoth attacks, and the like. They weren't designed for *chronic* heart weakening. Ultimately, these compensations turn out to be maladaptive. The rubber band stretches until it no longer has any spring. The fibers in the band initially thicken to get stronger, but eventually end up disordered, fibrotic, and useless.

The Starling compensation works for a while . . . until it doesn't. At some point, every CHF patient—as the medical shorthand puts it—falls off the Starling curve.

That morning, with russet autumn hues softening the Manhattan cityscape, with the incandescent optimism of a warm fall day pressing relentlessly into our small corner of the world, Julia teetered off the Starling curve.

—⁓—

It was eight years earlier that I'd first met Julia. She was thirty-five and healthy, cleaning bathrooms in an office building on the grave-yard shift to support her children. It wasn't her ideal job, but for an undocumented Guatemalan immigrant, it was the best she could get. She'd worked steadily until progressive shortness of breath had made it impossible to so much as lift a washcloth.

Julia was admitted to Bellevue Hospital with severe congestive heart failure. She landed on my ward only because my team happened to be up next when her admission was processed in the ER. Her CHF symptoms were quickly alleviated with diuretics and other medications, but there came the moment that we had to explain to her the full extent of her diagnosis. At that point, we knew she didn't have any reversible causes of CHF, that her heart was on a one-way course toward failure. Giving a difficult diagnosis to a patient is, of course, never easy. Emotions always run high—for doctors and patients alike.

But this moment was laced with an additional element of pain. Julia's failing heart could, in fact, be cured. A heart transplant is the standard treatment for otherwise healthy patients with irreversible CHF. Had Julia been born fifteen hundred miles farther north, we would have been discussing how she would get on the transplant list for new heart. But that's not what we would be telling her that morning. We were tasked, instead, with telling her that although her heart condition could be cured with a heart transplant, she could not get on the transplant list because she was undocumented.

We doctors were in an emotional bind. The rational doctor side of us knew exactly what facts to convey to her. But the emotional, human side of us could not bring ourselves to be the conveyers of this horrible twist of fate. To have a potential cure for your patient and then to have to tell your patient that she can't get it and will thus die places a human being in an emotionally untenable spot.

I first wrote about Julia in my book *Medicine in Translation* shortly after she plummeted off the Starling curve. We'd been together for eight intense years, and the fright of what might be the beginning of the end drove me to put pen to paper. The mere act of writing about her was a painful emotional experience, tracing the ups and downs of her medical roller coaster. But it was that first moment, trying to utter the actual words to her about her grim diagnosis and the impossibility of treatment, that was the hardest. I summarized that moment in an op-ed article about doctors and feelings.[1]

> It was a little bit like looking in the mirror. We were the same height and build, the same age—mid-30s—and both of us had two young children at home. In another world, had we been friends, we could have easily shared clothing. But today it was me with the white coat and her with the death sentence.
>
> Except she didn't know it yet.
>
> It was the morning of Julia's discharge from the hospital, and we were going through the array of cardiac medications stacked on her bedside table. She asked the same question about each bottle: "Will this medicine make my heart better?"
>
> I squirmed painfully around the question, weaving ever more elaborate explanations about controlling symptoms, enhancing breathing, minimizing fluid imbalances, improving exercise tolerance. I told every truth about every medication, but I could not bring myself to tell her the ultimate truth—that a roll of the genetic dice had doomed the fibrils of her heart, that her only chance was a heart transplant, that because she was an undocumented immigrant this was nigh impossible. That her children would grow up motherless.
>
> . . . When Julia walked out of our hospital without full knowledge of her prognosis, I had been derelict in my duty as her physician. I was fully aware that my job was to have "open and honest" communication with her, in a "patient-centered" manner. But I couldn't. I couldn't bring myself to tell this young mother that she was going to die.

It could be that I over-identified with my patient, or that I let my emotions get the better of me, or that I was an out-and-out wimp. No doubt all played some role, but I wasn't the only doctor who struggled with the truth. Everyone responsible for her care—intern, resident, medical attending, cardiology fellow, cardiology attending—independently fell short of the Charter on Medical Professionalism [that lists honest communication with patients as a paramount ethical pillar]. Young, old, male, female, touchy-feely, egotistical, blustery alike—not one of us could say those words to her face.

After this essay was published, the feedback was swift and furious. Many people excoriated me for not telling Julia the full truth of her diagnosis on that day. A common refrain was that I'd robbed her of time to process her diagnosis.

These critics were, of course, correct. I was wrong not to convey to her the extent of her predicament. I did rob her of time. But I wrote about this moment not solely to own up to my own shortcomings but to describe a situation in which emotions forcefully affect how doctors act, and how this impacts patients. I took some solace in the fact that every other doctor on the team was similarly incapacitated by this emotional conundrum. That observation of the universality of our reaction was part of what prompted me to write this book. None of us could escape it.

Julia did eventually get the truth of her diagnosis, at her first post-discharge clinic visit. The actual moment was—as expected—horrible. It took several tries for us to get the words on the table. Voices choked, eyes brimmed—and that was just the doctors. Julia was more stoic. She nodded slowly, very slowly, as she pieced it all together. The quiet that followed felt like a licking of the wounds for all parties. All wasn't sunny and optimistic, but there was a sense of reality, and now the planning could begin.

Why did it take us so long to tell her? It might have been that we doctors first had to come to terms with the diagnosis ourselves—however selfish that might sound. Perhaps, uncon-sciously, we were trying to give Julia breathing room. But all this may have been mere justification to make us feel better. The fact is that we didn't tell her the whole truth, up front, as we should have.

CHAPTER 2

Can We Build a Better Doctor?

No one questions whether empathy is important for medicine, but there is a debate as to whether empathy (or lack thereof) is innate or something that we learn along the road of life. It's clearly some combination of both, but it is intriguing to consider the relative contributions. Researchers in Italy did a fascinating experiment on empathy, using a video showing someone's hand getting pricked with a needle.[1]

The researchers postulated that they could document a biological empathic response by noting a change in neural activity in the area of the observer's brain that correlated to the spot on the hand in the video that was being pricked. That is, if you watched a needle enter the meat between the thumb and second finger, you felt pain in that area of your own hand, or at least in the part of your brain that represents that part of your hand. (If the hand in the video was rubbed gently with a Q-tip, there was no change in neural activity of the observer; it occurred only with pain.) This could constitute a neurologic equivalent of standing in another person's shoes.

On an initial written test, all the subjects scored high on empathy scales and showed no obvious racial bias. But when watching the videos, white subjects had a neurological reaction only when they saw white hands being stuck with a needle, and black subjects reacted only to black hands. Even though the subjects viewed themselves as empathic and nonracist on the written test, somehow their brains or their instincts betrayed them; they seemed to feel pain only when it occurred on hands similar to theirs.

But then the researchers did something unusual: they included a video of a hand that was dyed violet. This was a skin color different from both the black and the white subjects', and one the subjects had presumably never seen before. When the violet hand was punctured with a needle, both blacks and whites reacted.

This suggests that humans do have an ability, possibly innate, to empathize with people who appear different. However, somewhere along the line, we may unconsciously learn not to empathize with certain types of "others."

—⁓—

Smack square in this debate over whether empathy is innate or learned is the consistent and depressing observation that medical students seem to lose prodigious amounts of empathy as they progress along the medical training route.[2] Something in our medical training system serves to stamp out whatever empathy students bring with them on day one.

The research appears to conclude that it is the third year of the traditional medical curriculum that does the most damage. This is a dispiriting finding, as the third year of medical school is the one in which medical students take their first steps into actual patient care. For most students, the third year of medical school is eagerly awaited. After two long years sitting in classrooms, you get to actually *do* what it is that doctors do—be in hospitals, take care of patients. One would think that these first steps into real patient care would bring forth all the idealism that drove students to medical school in the first place—idealism that is sorely tested in the first two years of memorizing reams of arcane facts.

But the reverse seems to occur. After their seminal clinical experiences involving real contact with real patients, medical students emerge with their empathy battered. Their ideals of medicine as a profession are pummeled by their initiation into the real world of clinical medicine. And it is in this demoralized state that we send them into residency to accrue what are arguably the most influential and formative experiences of becoming practicing physicians.

Why do medical students lose empathy during the clinical years of medical school? There are likely many reasons. Some are related to the disorientation and fatigue experienced by students as they are thrown into the fire of hospital life—so different from the orderly, clean, controlled classroom life in which they have existed for two years. That student world is cemented along predetermined schedules, explicit curricula, definitive tests. Even if the knowledge requirements are overwhelming—as they are—medical students at least know what to expect, down to nearly every second of their waking hours.

Wednesday, 8:30 a.m.–10:00 a.m., Pathology class; Topic: Peptic Ulcer Disease, room 203, Professor O'Brien, pages 237–54 in *Robbins' Pathologic Basis of Disease*, Exam on December 15.

This elaborately structured world of lectures, labs, classrooms, tests, and professors is a heliotropic universe with the medical students squarely at the fiery center. Everything exists for their sake. Their medical education is the raison d'être of the entire enterprise.

When the students enter the wards, however, the tables are not just turned, they are upended entirely. Temperamentally, the world of the hospital is a different planet from the medical-school lecture hall. To the greenhorn, it is sheer anarchy. Some of this is the nature of medicine: human beings and their illnesses do not trouble themselves with schedules, flow charts, or textbooks.

Chemotherapy infusion protocols conflict with CT scanner availability, but bronchoscopy can only be done after the CT scan, however the pulmonologist was called away to an emergency so the bronchoscopy needs to be rescheduled. Mrs. Baradi spiked a fever so chemo needs to be canceled and the patient in the next bed over just developed an unusual rash so needs to be moved to an isolation room, but the ER is backed up with admissions so five new patients are coming to the ward at the same time and no isolation beds are available. Mr. Langley's family is here and needs to speak to his doctor, but 15-West is short-staffed today so two nurses will have to be "floated" over there, and if the ambulette forms aren't filled out immediately then Ms. Gemberson's discharge will be delayed another day. There's a code on 17-North—drop everything!

Hospital life—with its byzantine array of moving parts layered atop the unpredictable rhythms of illness—is a permanent state of flux. Seasoned doctors and nurses are accustomed to working with a certain amount of ongoing bedlam. But new medical students, used to the orderly scheduling of academic life, are overwhelmed. They are easy to spot on the wards, not just because of their short white coats but because of the befogged expressions on their faces as clinical medicine swirls around them. They stand awkwardly on the edges of the ward as people, stretchers, emergencies, hospital lingo, and rapidly changing clinical priorities zing past them at bewildering speeds.

To add to their discomfort, the students are astute enough to know that they don't actually have any real purpose on the wards, no definitive job description like the doctors, nurses, pharmacists, phlebotomists, respiratory therapists, X-ray technicians, clerks, orderlies, dietitians, housekeepers, and electricians. Medical students are there only to learn. The inherently self-centered nature of their existence in a setting that is not specifically designed for their education—as the classroom part of medical school had been—creates an intensely uncomfortable state of being.

They did choose a career in medicine to help others, didn't they? Most medical students desperately want to help out on the wards—to ease some of their guilt, to "pay back" the interns and residents who are teaching them, to do some good for the patients in need they see all around them. But it's hard to know where to start when your skills are minimal and everything is moving at breakneck speed with a paradoxically anarchic efficiency that you are sure to jam up. Indeed, the help that medical students earnestly offer often slows things down, a point that is painfully obvious to all parties involved.

Although medical students eventually acclimatize somewhat to the clinical tumult, most retain that awkward sense of feeling useless, of being a constant fifth wheel. This difficulty in finding purpose, in finding a justified place in the beehive, can cause many students to unconsciously curtail their desire for engagement and hence their empathy.

A second and perhaps even more significant factor in loss of empathy is what has been termed the hidden curriculum of medical school. The formal curriculum—what is taught in the lecture halls, what is embodied in the school's mission statement, what is intoned by the deans and senior faculty who usher the students into the sacred world of medicine—can be trounced in a thrice by the hidden or informal curriculum that the students are submerged in once they enter the clinical fray.

The students' true teachers are no longer the august, gray-haired professors who practiced medicine in "the days of the giants" but harried interns and residents in grubby white coats stained with the badges of medicine in the trenches. These younger doctors are the immediate interface with clinical medicine for the students. The students trail their interns and residents every waking minute and absorb from them how medicine is done—how it is spoken, thought, written, performed, attired, and equipped.

Residents and interns are the grunts of the medical profession, tasked, simply, with getting everything done. The practical side of the clinical buck stops with them (even if the ultimate clinical and legal responsibility rests with the attendings), and the house staff do whatever it takes to get everything done. With their scut lists in hand, their coat pockets doubling as supply cabinets, they are the embodiment of the pragmatic. While many still retain their interest in the theories and mechanisms of disease, the overriding modus operandi is utilitarian, because unlike the electricians, housekeepers, therapists, technicians, orderlies, dietitians, even the nurses and senior doctors, their job description has no bounds.

If an X-ray needs to be done and transport is not available, it is the intern who wheels the patient down to radiology. If a form needs to get to the social worker's office immediately because a discharge is riding on it but the fax machine is broken, there is the intern galloping down the stairs, paper in hand. Although house staff are not enamored of the clerical, administrative, transportation, and nonmedical miscellany that falls into their laps, they would rather do it themselves than suffer the time delays inherent in waiting for the regular channels to creak forward.

They don't want time delays for their patients because they do genuinely want the best, timeliest care for them. But they don't want time delays for themselves either, because time delays translate to more work. And more work translates to less sleep. (One doctor recalled a board game he and his colleagues used to play during residency. It was called the Intern Game. Instead of money, the units of the game were hours of sleep, and this is what you would "spend" for any activity or item in the game.)

There is a baseness to this, but it's the natural outcome of putting smart, competitive, perfectionist people in a high-stress system with myriads of ever-changing tasks for which they feel professional responsibility, coupled with sleep deprivation and the granite-hard fact of only twenty-four hours in the day . . . even in a sleepless one.

This whatever-it-takes-to-get-it-done attitude breeds an efficiency that often dispenses with niceties. This is not to say that every intern or resident is hopelessly callous and jaded. To the contrary, there is usually a deeply felt sense of personal responsibility that good house staff model for their students. But the primacy of pragmatism laced with gallows humor and ever-present physical exhaustion submerge the idealistic medical students in a decidedly unromantic view of medicine. The philosophical musings of Osler, Hippocrates, the deans, and the old-school attendings have little traction here.

The medical student observes that even the most thoughtful and humanistic intern operates under the brutal calculus that every minute spent on nonessentials simply prolongs the work. Sure, it's wonderful to have an in-depth conversation with a patient, to do a more thorough physical exam, to patiently explain the disease process to a family member, to read up on a rare disorder, to attend that lecture on communication skills, to visit a patient a third time in the day, to make those extra phone calls to unravel a patient's medical history, to let a patient ramble on without interruption—but none of these will get the work done. The scut list will still be there.

In the first two years of medical school, every student in the class has the same educational experience. They all have the same lectures, the same professors, the same labs. For better or worse, it's relatively uniform. Once on the wards, though, it is a roll of the dice. The students are divvied up to different hospitals, different wards, different medical teams. For each student, it may come down to the individual intern he or she is paired with that makes or breaks the experience. If he is lucky and gets a fantastic intern who takes the time to teach and who treats the medical student with respect, the student will have a rewarding experience. If the student is assigned to an intern who is overwhelmed or jaded or derogatory toward patients, the student will end up with a decidedly different view of medicine.

I once supervised a group of medical students in Israel who were pressing through their third-year clerkships. We met monthly to discuss their progress, and each was required to hand in a few paragraphs about the experience. As I read through their comments about ob-gyn, I was amazed to see the polarized responses. One student wrote about how she surprised herself by falling in love with the field. Her team took her to every delivery. She helped out during cesarean sections. They let her be the first of the team to interview new patients so she could make the initial assessment. Though she came to medical school thinking she wanted to become a pediatrician, now ob-gyn was on her list as a career to consider.

The student whose essay followed hers couldn't think of enough awful things to say about ob-gyn. For his entire rotation, he mainly stood around doing nothing. His team was so busy that they hardly noticed him. By the time someone remembered to tell him about a fascinating case, the baby was already delivered and the action was over. He was viewed as an impediment and so he withdrew to the library, spending most of his time reading textbooks. He was so bitter that he couldn't possibly imagine himself ever going into ob-gyn.

Thus, whatever the medical student has been taught, and even genuinely believes, about the ideals of medicine, the primacy of empathy, the value of the doctor-patient relationship—all of this is swamped once he or she steps into the wards. Even the most idealistic student can start to view every new admission as an additional burden, every patient's request as another obstacle to getting the work done, every moment of casual conversation as a moment less of sleep. It's no wonder that empathy gets trounced in the actual world of clinical medicine; everything that empathy requires seems to detract from daily survival.

—ᨆ—

One of the most significant things that medical students are exposed to when they enter the clinical world is the language of medicine. These students arrive on the wards speaking normal, everyday English and are promptly immersed in the peculiar dialect of medicine. (Many leave residency training hardly able to string a noun, verb, and adjective together to make a normal sentence!) Some of this is simply shorthand, and it is particularly pronounced in the written chart.

A typical first line of a hospital admission might read *82 WM w/ PMH of CAD, CVA, MIx2, s/p 3V-CABG, c/o CP, SOB 2 wks PTA. BIBA s/p LOC. No F/C/N/V/D.* To the naïve medical student—and the rest of the human race—this is unintelligible. To any doctor, this is a perfectly succinct seventy-four-character description of an eighty-two-year-old white male with a past medical history of coronary artery disease, stroke, two heart attacks, and a triple-vessel cardiac-bypass operation who had complained of chest pain and shortness of breath for two weeks prior to admission. He was brought in by ambulance after loss of consciousness. He had no fever, chills, nausea, vomiting, or diarrhea. (This version in regular English—in case you were counting—took 309 characters.)

In addition to medical shorthand, there is the host of medical terminology to learn. A student has to become conversant in xerostomia, volvulus, sideroblastosis, fluoroscopy, choledocholithiasis, borborygmi, tenesmus, ileocolitis, Roux-en-Y, polycythemia vera, and palpable purpura. This can be very disorienting to new medical students, who are still trying to figure out where the bathrooms are.

On the flip side, this is what makes medical students the best allies for the patients. The students know what it's like to be struggling in this foreign medical language and are usually the most generous and helpful in interpreting the alien terminology for the patient and family.

Beyond all of the "proper" medical linguistics, however, there is the hospital slang that comes with the territory. More than anything else, slang seems to be the most potent indicator that one is a full-fledged member of the tribe, and medical students are highly attuned to the vernacular that permeates the clinical world. Some of this slang can be benign, or even self-deprecating, such as when an orthopedist refers to himself as a bonehead or radiologists joke about hiding out in their cave (darkened room for reading X-rays).

But much of the slang and gallows humor can be rather derogatory, especially with regard to patients. A whining Central American patient—like Maríssima Alvarez—is diagnosed with "status Hispanicus," a play on status asthmaticus, which is a prolonged, overwhelming asthma attack. A surly, uncooperative drug addict is "not a citizen"; this has nothing to do with immigrants, and everything to do with the human race.

These derogatory terms, by definition, serve to distance doctor from patient, and this directly detracts from the ability to be empathic. While some of this slang seems merely callous, a lot of it derives from fear. Some of the states in which our patients live—or die—are downright terrifying. To empathize with these patients, to put yourself in their shoes, may be a bit too existentially disconcerting. And so doctors unconsciously try to protect themselves by widening the moat between their own good health and their patients' dauntingly mortal conditions. Hence, an elderly, demented, incontinent, babbling patient from a nursing home is a "gomer" or is "gorked out." A dying patient is "circling the drain."

Medical students want desperately to be in the club, to appear seasoned, to seem competent; medical slang and inside jokes are a way of achieving this. Not knowing slang is the clearest indication of a newbie.

I once listened to a determinedly thorough case presentation from a brand-new medical student. It was his first day on the medical service and he was presenting the case of a patient who had been admitted the night before. The admission note had been written by the overnight intern, and the medical student was following that intern's notes as best he could. The student negotiated most of the intern's shorthand, but then he got to the GU (genitourinary) exam.

Embryologically, the testes begin life inside the pelvis, and then they descend into the scrotum, where they spend the rest of their days in this pleasantly cooler environment that is more conducive to sperm production. On a routine physical exam, a physician palpates the scrotum to check that both have descended, because an undescended testicle might require surgical correction. The standard intern notation to indicate that both testes are appropriately descended is ↓↓ *testes* and is read aloud as "bilaterally descended testes." The student, who was reading along smoothly by this point and starting to gain confidence, stated—without missing a beat—"The patient had extremely small testes."

The rest of the team, who had been listening politely up until then, was unable to hold back and erupted in laughter. The student—who had already moved on to reading aloud the details of rectal exam—snapped his head up at the laughter, entirely perplexed. He had no idea what was funny.

When someone finally told him that those two down-going arrows meant "bilaterally descended," not "extremely small," he reddened like a late-summer cherry tomato. It was not just the mistake that embarrassed him; it was that his ignorance of the medical shorthand (which everyone else so plainly knew) had pinned him as the greenhorn that he was, setting him apart from the "real" doctors, who decoded this language effortlessly.

Medical students devote significant attention—even if unconsciously—to discerning what they need to absorb in order to look and sound like real doctors. They note not only how the attending palpates the spleen but also whether her white coat is buttoned or unbuttoned, whether the clothes underneath are casual or business attire. They glean subtle messages from even the most mundane details, such as whether the stethoscope is draped around the neck (the cocky announcement of a doctor who lives only in the pragmatic present, ferociously occupied with saving lives) or sitting coolly curled in the pocket, edges peeking out (the understated ID card of one who is running the show but doesn't necessarily need to blare that out).

Students incorporate their superiors' manner of interaction with nurses, administrators, patients, and family members. They assimilate proper medical grammar that is as exquisitely precise as Latin declensions. Hence, the patient "endorses fatigue, but denies dyspnea" (as opposed to "the patient is tired, but not short of breath"). Among all of this vast medical and sociological learning, the students also divine what sort of slang and humor is acceptable and what is not.

Medical students' reactions to jokes have been a surprisingly fruitful area of research.[3] It turns out that there are complex rules for the "humor game," never verbalized but universally agreed upon. Only the most senior physician can initiate joking, for example, and that person sets the acceptability meter for humorous banter; no joke can go beyond the line drawn by the most senior doctor's joke. There are specific places that are okay for joking—hallways, conference rooms, areas perceived to be private. Joking is verboten in elevators and patient rooms.

There are unspoken but clear rules for acceptable targets: drug abusers are okay; cancer patients are not. Alcoholism and obesity are okay; miscarriage is not. Schizophrenic and borderline patients—yes; terminally ill patients—no. And children with cancer—never.

For medical students, this slang and humor puts them in a bind. By dint of being in the white coat, they are insiders, so privy to this, but mostly they still feel like outsiders. They cringe at the crassness of the language, often feel disgusted, but they are laboring to be insiders and feel they must nod in agreement to such jokes. Or they unwittingly absorb it, as they instinctively model their superiors. Empathy-sapping terminology like *gomer* and *not a citizen* and *circling the drain* trickle down quickly and unconsciously from senior doctors and residents to the students.

Despite sometimes feeling repulsed by the jokes, medical students—and senior doctors too—sense that the humor is not actually mean-spirited, or at least not intended to be. They see the humor as directed at the situation rather than at the patient (though it's hard to imagine a patient sharing that perspective were she to overhear). Physicians of all levels tend to explain black humor in terms of defusing stress and dealing with impossible situations. An ICU physician known for his biting humor once told me, "Everyone in here is dying. What else can you do but joke?"

For doctors, as for all people, humor can be a reflexive a way of dealing with personal discomfort. Children are notorious for smiling and giggling when they are being reprimanded. Medical personnel, likewise, can react with seemingly inappropriate humor in awkward circumstances.

Doctors at any level—but especially students and trainees—can feel overwhelmed in certain situations, sometimes entirely powerless. There are many ways more constructive than humor to handle these emotions, but often we aren't able to access them, at least in the moment. I have a crystal-clear recollection of my first night in the psychiatric emergency room at Bellevue. If Bellevue's ER is the belly of the beast, then its psychiatric ER is the colonic innards of that belly—the stuff of legend, TV sitcoms, and late-night comedians.

I was a third-year medical student taking my first steps on the wards. Unlike other third-years—whose clinical rotations follow on the heels of their basic-science years—I'd been out of the loop for a significant chunk of time. Because I did my PhD between the first and second halves of medical school, I'd been closeted away in the lab for nearly four years, immersed in the research side of medical science where the most belligerent thing I had to deal with was pipettes that jammed. My days were lined with the crisp serenity of experimental design and hypothesis testing. I would start each day smoothing out rows of immaculate test tubes, the faint friction of the polystyrene yielding easily to my fingers. Each and every variable of the experiment was mine to control.

From this orderly world of empiricism and rational thought, I segued straight into the Bellevue psych ER. At the time, the psych ER was a grubby side room off the main ER. A single narrow door led into a cramped, windowless waiting room. There were three closet-size rooms for interviewing patients in private, but for the most part everyone dwelt in that waiting room—patients, residents, students, nurses, and orderlies. It was here that cops brought in the craziest of New York City's crazy. Often these patients were homeless, usually as a result of their psychiatric conditions, often in conjunction with their drug and alcohol use. A colossal black police officer hovered at the door, keeping a wary eye on everything and everyone. His imposing width and breadth, and especially his prodigious height, obliterated the doorway, as well as any hope of escape. When I edged passed him into the waiting room, I barely cleared his holster.

Beyond being chaotic in sight and sound, the waiting room of the psych ER stank. The lack of ventilation, the close proximity of bodies, and the generally unshowered state of the patients combined to give the place a permanent pungency. It was like the smell I'd encountered years earlier with the rape victim, only magnified tenfold by the number of patients in the cramped space. The staff barely seemed to notice, but for the uninitiated it was overwhelming.

I was an uninitiated to the nth degree—I hadn't so much as laid eyes on a patient of any sort in years—and my gears shifted into a sudden and perpetual state of nausea. The disgusting smell wormed its way inside me, eliciting the same reaction I'd had as a first-year student in the emergency room, and I couldn't imagine how I was going to spend the next twelve hours in this confined space.

The patient who I'd been assigned to interview was a young white woman, maybe in her twenties. She'd been found half naked in the subway, delusional and violent, in the throes of a psychotic break. Evidently she'd still been combative in the ER despite sedation, because she was now in four-point restraints. She was a wisp of a figure on the stretcher, looking both pathetic and terrifying. Her psychotic spiral had been progressing for some time, it seemed, because she'd acquired the grime and rancid odor of living on the street.

The resident I was working with seemed to intuit my discomfort. He had curly golden-brown hair that swooped seamlessly into a full beard and mustache, making him look biblical, despite his raggedy blue scrubs, which were the preferred attire of everyone working overnight at Bellevue, from orderlies to surgeons to psychiatrists. He pulled me into one of the tiny rooms and closed the door. "Don't worry," he said. "It's only toxic sock syndrome. It comes with the territory."

Maybe it was just being in ground zero of insanity in the middle of the night with someone who looked right out of *The Ten Commandments,* but I burst out laughing. I'd never heard the term *toxic sock syndrome* before, and it struck me as hysterical, even as I saw that it was derogatory toward our patient. But I couldn't help myself. Somehow it encapsulated the situation so penetratingly. I broke down in full-throated belly laughs, and it took several minutes for me to regain my composure.

When I finally followed Dr. Moses back out to the waiting room, I found myself better able to tolerate the smell. It was still sharp and bothersome, but I was somehow able to push it aside in my consciousness. I remained aware of the odor during all my time in the ER, but it no longer overwhelmed me.

When I tried to interview the young woman, however, she wouldn't answer my questions. She would only say, "I need the bathroom. You gotta untie me. I need the bathroom." I, of course, was petrified. I didn't want her to wet her pants, but I didn't know if I was allowed to undo the restraints. "You gotta untie me," she kept intoning. "You gotta untie me."

Moses had disappeared into another exam room, so I tiptoed over to one of the nurses for help. The nurse heaved a sigh and plastered me with one of those looks; a veteran nurse can take down a medical student with no more than a blink. "She's really got to pee," I begged. The nurse walked over to the patient and asked her a battery of questions, then reluctantly undid the restraints and helped the patient to her feet.

The patient hovered unsteadily for a moment, then slowly regained her sea legs. Standing up, she looked even scrawnier than when she'd been lying down. If she clocked in at a hundred pounds, I'd be impressed. She sauntered across the waiting room, but instead of going to the bathroom, she went over to the cop who was guarding the entrance. She looked up at him—a distance of probably two feet. "Hey, N-word," she said by way of pleasant greeting. At the same time, she reached out her hand and grabbed his crotch, squeezing with staggering strength. As the two-hundred-and-seventy-pound cop crumpled to the floor like a sack of cement, the patient turned and casually continued toward the bathroom.

Thus transpired day one for me in the Bellevue psych ER. To say it was overwhelming would be beyond understatement. But I've since thought a lot about why I laughed so hard at the toxic-sock-syndrome crack. It was a crude, derogatory joke. As an attending now, I'd probably take an intern to task if I overheard him say it. But in retrospect, I can see that my reaction, perhaps overreaction, to the resident's joke had more to do with my discomfort and my sense of utter bewilderment than his innate comedic skills. I'm not proud of colluding with the resident at the expense of our patient—who, thankfully, couldn't hear us—but with distance I can better understand how it occurred. I also remember that I felt differently about myself after that aside. Having been confided in, trusted with an inside joke, I was now part of the team—an insider rather than an outsider.

It makes me wonder if humor could be a teaching tool in and of itself. Not that I am advocating inserting sarcastic jokes into the curriculum, but the experience does give me pause. I try to envision sitting in a lecture on how to deal with horrible smells. It's hard to imagine that it would offer much help. But the joke seemed to release something inside me, something unconscious that allowed me to step into this difficult situation. I was even able to consider the smell something poignant, something that spoke to the patient's suffering. Now when I enter a room with that kind of smell, I still get the visceral discomfort, but it doesn't incapacitate me. It actually heightens my awareness of the patient's vulnerability. It reminds me to take extra care, as that nurse's aide did with the rape victim, so many years back.

—⁂—

All through my medical training, I avoided reading *The House of God* because I knew that it was derogatory, sexist, dated, and downright offensive. When I was invited to contribute to a commemorative anthology celebrating the twenty-fifth anniversary of Samuel Shem's now-classic book, I had to politely decline, since (I was abashed to admit) I hadn't read it. At which point I figured I ought to go ahead and crack the cover, if only because it had become a cultural icon.

The book was everything that I'd expected—derogatory, sexist, dated, offensive. But for four hundred pages I laughed so hard that people nearby thought I was having seizures. The book went against nearly everything I valued, yet for the life of me, I could not stop laughing. I was embarrassed at how funny I found the book.

But like the toxic-sock-syndrome joke that somehow got me beyond my gag reflex with awful smells, there were parts of the book the drove to the heart of difficult issues through humor.

There is a scene in *The House of God* in which the intern Roy is faced with an unresponsive elderly patient in room 116 named Anna O. (who is, of course, duly referred to as a gomer). He is sure that she is dead, since she won't answer him, and he can't find a pulse or a heartbeat.

"Oh, she looks dead, sure. I'll give you that," says the resident known as the Fat Man. "With Anna, you need the reverse stethoscope technique. Watch."

> The Fat Man took off his stethoscope, plugged the earpiece into Anna O.'s ears, and then, using the bell like a megaphone, shouted into it: "Cochlea come in, cochlea come in, do you read me, cochlea come . . ."
>
> Suddenly the room exploded. Anna O. was rocketing up and down on the stretcher, shrieking at great pitch and intensity.

The image of a resident hollering into the bottom of the stethoscope trying to communicate with a demented patient is obviously demeaning when you think about the patient, who is somebody's sister or mother. But when you think about it in terms of the immense frustration and overwhelming sense of helplessness that interns feel when they care for patients with severe dementia who don't talk or respond in any way, you can get a sense of why this resonates. The Fat Man yelling into the stethoscope to wake up Anna O. is absurd, yet it brings forward the challenges in a way that a PowerPoint slide could never match. As satire, it allows you to laugh at yourself as the bumbling doctor who feels like an utter idiot trying to communicate with a severely demented patient.

Reading this scene, I found myself empathizing with the intern, but also with Anna O. It gave me a feeling for how distant she'd grown from herself, of how dementia had elbowed away the person she once was. The silliness of the scene itself had a poignancy. In a counterintuitive way, it underscored both her humanity and that of the struggling intern. It reminded me of my first night in the psych ER, and how both the patient and I were grappling—if imperfectly—with frightening, disorienting situations.

In the early days of AIDS, when the disease was more mysterious and far more terrifying than it is today, jokes and slang abounded. HIV patients with fevers—every other patient, it seemed, when I was a resident—were HIVers with shivers. HIV-positive gay men who continued to have unprotected sex were AIDS terrorists. There were tattoo algorithms, which allowed you to calculate the probability that the HIV test would come back positive based on the number of tattoos you found on your patient during the physical exam. And there were the AIDS dice that sat in the doctors' station of 17-West, the AIDS ward at Bellevue. No one remembered who had created these dice, made from wadded-up surgical tape, but there next to the X-ray light box sat the pair—one for diagnosis and one for prognosis.

The diagnosis die was labeled with the common diseases that AIDS patients were admitted for: PCP, CMV, MAI, KS, NHL, TB (pneumocystis pneumonia, cytomegalovirus, mycobacterium avium-intracellulare, Kaposi's sarcoma, non-Hodgkin's lymphoma, and tuberculosis, respectively). The prognosis die contained shorthand for the various outcomes available to AIDS patients in the 1990s: DNR, ICU, ECU, 12-E. The extended-care unit—ECU—was slang for death; 12-East was the spillover ward where we moved patients who were imminently dying (12-East had private rooms—a rarity for Bellevue. Needless to say, 12-East was always full).

As soon as your pager went off signaling a new admission in the emergency room, you'd quickly roll the dice and note which diagnosis and which prognosis came up. Then you would dash to the ER to admit your patient. If the diagnosis/prognosis of the dice was a perfect match to the new patient, you "won" for that night.

In retrospect, the AIDS dice were crude, cynical, and demeaning. At the time, though, they struck us as not only harmless fun but also oddly appropriate. AIDS itself was a crapshoot in life. Why *not* just roll the dice?

The 1990s was an immensely depressing time for medical training. HIV saturated our lives in a way that is hard for me to describe to my own students now. Witnessing one's own generation dying off is not for the faint of heart. The gallows humor that flowed at this time was related to this overwhelming tide of death but also to our own existential fears. I don't think we were aware how much this distanced us from our patients and challenged our ability to be empathic.

There were no doubt more sophisticated ways of dealing with our feelings than the AIDS dice and the ongoing black humor—certainly ways that would have been less demeaning to our patients—but there wasn't much touchy-feely guidance available for residents then. And there certainly wasn't any spare time for it; the minute an AIDS patient was discharged or died, another one was zipped up from the ER, where patients in gurneys lined the hallways awaiting beds in the wards. The cycle of illness and death pelted along mercilessly. There was little time to breathe, much less reflect or contemplate.

Earlier in the epidemic, before even the basics of AIDS were understood, fear and discomfort were even stronger. I was a first-year medical student in 1986, when the HIV virus was still called HTLV-III and the first AIDS drug—AZT—hadn't yet been approved by the FDA. A joke circulated among the class of nervous first-years: "What's the worst part about telling your parents that you have AIDS?" Answer: "Explaining to them that you are a Haitian immigrant."

Almost everyone in my predominantly white and Asian medical school class thought this was a witty joke, encapsulating how we could never admit to being gay or taking drugs, and subliminally encompassing our fears of this baffling, gruesome, and untreatable epidemic. And we, of course, unconsciously clung to the hope that being white or Asian upper-middle-class medical students would protect us.

The joke itself quickly became laughable, since Haitian immigrants ceased to be a high-risk group almost immediately. Over the subsequent two decades, AIDS receded into an "ordinary" chronic disease not nearly as mysterious and uniformly fatal as it once was. The AIDS service at Bellevue closed down for lack of acutely ill patients. The 17-West AIDS ward became a regular medical ward. The 12-East dying ward was turned into offices. The disease moved to the outpatient setting to take its place next to diabetes, hypertension, and other prosaic chronic afflictions that fill the past-medical-history boxes of our patients' charts. As a profession and as a society, we acclimatized to AIDS. As a result, the jokes and slang largely faded. The AIDS dice disappeared during renovations.

—⁓—

We see an array of factors that ambush the empathy that students enter medical school with—the hidden curriculum, derogatory humor, mixed messages from residents, fatigue, and the sheer overwhelming nature of it all. The question then arises: Does this have to be a given? That is, does the system designed to train doctors have to be an empathy-sapping experience?

Researchers have been asking whether it is possible to prevent this documented decline in empathy during medical school. All sorts of suggestions have been offered: medical humanities, flexible scheduling, reflective writing, role-playing, additional vacation, faculty mentoring, nutritious lunches, peer-support groups, earlier clinical exposure. Many of these things are hard to test in the typical rigorous scientific manner that is expected of any medical intervention. Mostly, these proposed solutions come from observational studies, personal philosophies, inspiration, and perhaps wishful thinking.

To actually study empathy—its decline and perhaps the prevention thereof—one first needs to be able to measure empathy in an objective manner. This may seem counterintuitive, empathy being the sort of thing most people know when they see, but a true scientific study can be done only with numbers, not feelings. And so, a numerical measure of empathy was created.

A group of researchers at Jefferson Medical College in Philadelphia created the deceptively simple Jefferson Scale of Empathy (JSE),[4] a single page containing twenty statements, each to be rated from 1 (strongly disagree) to 6 (strongly agree). Their definition of empathy is specifically distinct from sympathy. For the researchers, sympathy is an emotion, actually feeling the patient's feelings. Empathy is a cognition, a thought process that allows you to understand the patient's feelings while not necessarily feeling them yourself. In fact, maintaining your own sense of self is a key part of empathy. The empathy definition might thus be reworded as the ability to stand in another's shoes without actually leaving your own shoes. And of course the empathic doctor needs to be able to clearly communicate that understanding (i.e., it's not empathy if the patient doesn't realize your understanding of his or her feelings).[5]

The statements on the JSE appear relatively straightforward, in the sense that most medical students would seem to know what they are "supposed to" strongly agree with or strongly disagree with:

> *Patients feel better when their physicians understand their feelings.*

> *Physicians should try to stand in their patients' shoes when providing care to them.*

> *I believe that empathy is an important therapeutic factor in medical treatment.*

or

> *I believe that emotion has no place in the treatment of medical illness.*

> *Asking patients about what is happening in their personal lives is not helpful in understanding their physical complaints.*

Patients' illnesses can be cured only by medical or surgical treatment; therefore physicians' emotional ties with their patients do not have a significant influence.

Medical students by this stage in their academic careers are extremely adept at saying what they think their superiors want to hear, and one would think that they'd all mark strongly agree next to the top three "correct" statements and strongly disagree next to the second triad of "incorrect" statements.

Surprisingly, at least to me, the scale does seem to tease out different slivers of students. Those who score higher on the empathy scale go on to choose people-oriented specialties (primary care, pediatrics, psychiatry), whereas those who score lower tend toward procedure-oriented specialties (surgery, radiology, anesthesiology). High empathy scores predict which students will excel in their clinical clerkships, who will be nominated by their peers for exemplary professionalism, and who will be ranked as highly empathic by residency program directors and by patients themselves.[6]

Armed with a tool that appears to measure empathy, researchers could quantitate the decline in empathy and then study interventions to try to prevent this seemingly inevitable erosion.

In one study at Robert Wood Johnson Medical School in New Jersey, students participated in a Humanism and Professionalism Program during the course of their third year.[7] The program was a joint creation of students and faculty that involved a one-hour meeting during each of the six required rotations (surgery, medicine, pediatrics, ob-gyn, psychiatry, and family medicine). With faculty facilitators, the students discussed the tribulations of patient care, difficult situations they faced, burnout, positive and negative role models they were exposed to, and the specific challenges of maintaining humanism and professionalism in situations that often seemed expressly designed to chip away at these values. Students also posted blog entries about their experiences, which turned out to be important triggers for discussion. Additionally, students were given readings—from both doctors and patients—that reflected upon experiences in medicine.

Two consecutive classes of medical students took the JSE before they started this program in their third year and then again at the end of the year. On average, the researchers found no decline in empathy scores for both classes, which led them to conclude that this sort of intensive discussion/reading/awareness might be able to prevent the dreaded third-year slump.

The main limitation of the study, of course, was that there was no direct control group. They didn't divide the class in two and allow only one half to participate in the program. Nor did they administer the same test to the previous classes, who didn't have the benefit of the program. However, the empathy scores of these incoming third-year students were the same as those of third-year students in studies I cited earlier. The students in the other studies showed the decline after they finished their clinical rotations, but the students who took the Humanism and Professionalism course in this study did not.

Educators at the University of California at San Francisco and at Harvard took a different approach. Rather than enrich the students with humanities in an attempt to "inoculate" them against the battering effects of the third year of medical school, they decided to scrap the third year altogether and create something new. They noted that the traditional clerkships (four to eight weeks each) resulted in a revolving-door frenzy of students cycling in and out of hospitals, wards, teams, and patients' lives. How could anyone maintain focus—much less sanity—when every ounce of stability was upended with brutal regularity? How could a medical student, already in a daze in this bizarre hospital world, find any depth of relationship with patients, colleagues, and mentors? Such "enforced transientness" is deleterious to empathy for patients and the psychological well-being of caregivers, and it can also result in disastrous medical care for patients.[8]

The faculty decided to dispense with the rotational craziness, and instead they created a full-year program that sought to integrate all the medical specialties. The students would have a "home" from which they could participate in many aspects of the hospital world. This would give the students the ability to follow patients long-term, through critical illness in the hospital, at outpatient visits after discharge, even at home visits.

Students might follow a pregnant woman through pregnancy, attend the delivery, then continue with the pediatrics visits of the baby. Students might care for a terminally ill patient in the hospital, follow the patient in hospice, and even continue meeting with the family after the patient's death. There would be a single faculty mentor for each student throughout the clinical experience to provide stability, though the students would still have the opportunity to work with a variety of other attendings in different practice settings.

While this is a new approach in urban and suburban medicine, it has been a staple of rural medicine, where doctors care for patients of all ages and typically stay involved over the course of a lifetime. At the University of Minnesota Medical School, students can spend a full year living, working, and learning in a rural setting.

There is no doubt that such a program is much more complicated to arrange than the traditional rotation-based training. There is far more logistical coordination required, but the real financial cost is the tremendous amount of faculty involvement required. (From the medical center's perspective, any hour an attending physician diverts from direct patient care to teaching is lost revenue. This becomes the bottom-line calculation for these programs.)

This integrated approach was studied formally at Harvard Medical School, where a group of students in the integrated clerkship were compared with the rest of the class who followed the traditional path of rotating clerkships.[9] In terms of academic achievement and clinical skills, there was no difference between the students. But the students in the integrated clerkship scored higher in analyses of how they approached ethical dilemmas and how they helped patients and families with complex decision-making; 100 percent of them felt that they had established meaningful relationships with patients, compared with 55 percent of students in the traditional model. The students in the first group were far more comfortable in dealing with ambiguity and more willing to reflect on their own weaknesses and strengths. And in the overall analysis, they were much happier with their educational experience and felt that their ideals about medicine had been preserved.

To me, these studies transcend the question of whether medical schools should teach empathy or simply select students who already have empathy. In fact, we need to do both. The traditional entrance exam for medical school, the MCAT, is being overhauled to contain sections on ethics, philosophy, humanities, and social sciences.[10] While this doesn't guarantee students with empathy skills, it certainly widens the focus beyond organic chemistry. And programs that enrich students with humanities, long-term patient contact, and one-on-one mentoring can help minimize ethical erosion and other toxic effects of medical school.

The truth is that most students enter medical school with strong humanistic and empathic tendencies. Having worked with hundreds of medical students over the years, I know firsthand that these characteristics are not in short supply. The challenge for medical schools is to maintain and nourish these qualities during the long haul of training.

Unlike pathophysiology, however, none of this can be taught in lecture halls or with PowerPoint slides. It is the behaviors that students witness in their superiors and the behaviors that are modeled and encouraged that really count, and luckily, the new approaches of medical schools are focusing on this.

My analogy for teaching empathy is that of multiculturalism. This topic is very politically correct these days; medical schools and hospitals are scrambling to offer cultural-sensitivity seminars and culture-awareness days. These programs tend to be well meaning, extremely earnest, and only marginally useful.

What influences my own clinical practice are the lessons I received from a cadre of older, white, male physicians—my own attendings—who wore starched shirts, conservative ties (often of the bow variety), and properly buttoned white coats to every clinical encounter. They trained in an era in which their entire medical-school class looked exactly like them, with no diversity awareness, affirmative action, or cultural competence.

Yet they were among the most culturally aware people I've ever seen, though they probably would never use such a PC term. These physicians exemplified a very old-fashioned sort of doctoring. For them, approaching the bedside of a patient was a sacred act. They examined each patient—whether a homeless Ecuadoran alcoholic or a veiled Muslim woman or a visiting Swiss diplomat—with a thoroughness that in itself exuded respect. They asked questions to learn more and listened with an exacting ear, for the axiom that the patient's story holds the answers was no platitude for them.

What these older physicians exhibited is termed *clinical curiosity*. They strove to understand their patients in order to elucidate the underlying medical conditions. This thoroughness, patience, and dogged curiosity may have been ingrained in them because they trained at a time when there were no rapid CTs or MRIs. But even now, when these diagnostic tools are at their fingertips, these physicians maintain this approach to patients, one that serves to appreciate the dignity and uniqueness of each patient and his or her illness.

I doubt if any of these physicians ever backpacked in Nepal or worked for the Peace Corps in Uganda or campaigned for human rights in Honduras or took any multicultural-awareness workshops. They simply treated every patient with respect, and strove to learn as much as possible about each one.

I can recall rounding with them at Bellevue when I was a student, thinking how out of place these starched white men looked in a ward full of Hispanics, Asians, and blacks; how different their educated backgrounds were from these patients who were often poor, uneducated recent immigrants. I expected these doctors to form only a limited connection with these patients because of the vast socioeconomic and cultural divide. Similarly, I expected the patients to be uncomfortable, perhaps intimidated by these white male figures of authority.

But it was quite the opposite. When these doctors treated the patients with old-school respect, exhibiting genuine curiosity about their lives, the patients responded wholeheartedly. I marveled at these older male physicians who asked such nuanced and probing questions about culture and background. In this manner, these physicians were demonstrating empathy. The very act of taking a patient and her story seriously, of being truly interested in knowing who the patient is and what her life is like and how she came to be ill and what her resources for dealing with illness were, is the basis of empathy.

Teaching empathy to medical students and interns falls not to the course directors who devise the curriculum and establish the core competencies but to the supervising doctors who oversee these trainees on the wards. Students will remember what they experience far better than what they are told in a lecture, as I learned those many years ago watching that nurse's aide help the homeless woman in the ER.

Astute clinical teachers also explicitly point out to students what they do and say with patients to help convey empathy. Even tiny tips, like reminding students to summarize what a patient has said and offer it back for corrections, is helpful. When a doctor says, "Let me see if I have this right . . . ," it indicates to a patient that the doctor is not only listening hard but also making an effort to understand the patient's point of view.[11]

One month into medical school, I and a few other nervous first-year students were ushered into the office of Dr. Frank Spencer to learn how to interview patients. Dr. Spencer, a cardiothoracic surgeon who pioneered cardiac bypass surgery and repair of bleeding arteries, had a fearsome, Texas-size reputation in the hospital. Residents and students quaked when he interrogated them about patient care. I once (some years later) witnessed him berate a resident in front of the entire department during an M&M—the infamous Morbidity and Mortality rounds in which errors and bad outcomes are reviewed. Referring to what he regarded as substandard care, he sniped in his languid, marbles-in-the-mouth Texan twang: "If you're gonna practice medicine like that, why bother operatin' on the patient at all? Just take him outside with a rifle and shoot the man already."

But patients worshipped him. And I quickly learned why. For starters, his bluster was not about denigrating and humiliating residents (though some certainly felt that way) but about demanding top-notch care for every single patient and not settling for one iota less. Patients keyed into this quickly and knew that Dr. Spencer would fight tooth and nail for them. But what he taught me in his exam room that first meeting gave me another insight.

Wordlessly, he dragged a low metal stool from the side of the room over to the exam table while we students flattened ourselves against the wall and watched. The stool was swiveled down to its lowest height and when he sat himself down on it, his head was about at the level of the exam table. "Whenever you talk to a patient," he said, "you seat yourself at their level or lower. You never hover over them high and mighty. They are the ones who are sick, and they are the ones running this interview, not you."

It was a simple gesture, but it spoke volumes about how he approached a patient. For me, as a student grappling with what kind of doctor I wanted to be, it was a powerful moment. If this commanding doctor at the top of the heap had no issues about being humble with a patient, then it was okay to do. As I wended my way through my medical training, I observed what my superiors said and how they acted with patients. And I watched how patients responded and could tell what worked (and what didn't). Not all of my teachers were as explicit as Dr. Spencer, but they were teaching—even if unconsciously—every second of the day.

When I interviewed Dr. Spencer more than twenty-five years after our initial meeting, he hadn't changed much at all. Nattily dressed and chivalrous, with perceptive eyes and a nearly unlined face, he held court in his meticulous office that was covered with photos and memorabilia from his Korean War service. A black-and-white photo showed a lone mesquite tree set against a vast stretch of empty field. He was born fifty feet from that tree, he told me, and was raised in a ranching and farming family.

What he remembers most about his military service was being shocked the first time he saw a soldier with a bleeding femoral artery get treated with ligation (tying off) of the artery and then subsequent amputation of the leg when he knew that it was possible to surgically repair the artery and save the leg. The army surgeons opened the field manual and showed him the page that dictated ligation treatment for bleeding arteries.

Frank gathered his medic buddies and announced that he was going to start repairing these arteries, not ligating them, even though it was against regulations. He convinced his fellow medics to go along with him. "We'll either get medals of valor or court-martialed," he told them. They defied army regulations, and as a result, hundreds of soldiers returned home from Korea with two legs instead of one. The medal of valor hangs on his wall next to the photo of the mesquite tree.

Frank Spencer struck me as, if anything, even more devoted now to connecting with patients, and he felt that most patients' anger at physicians and the resultant lawsuits stem from the doctors' lack of empathy and genuine communication.

When I brought up Osler's "Aequanimitas," about doctors keeping an emotional distance from patients, he gave a snort of derision. "Garbage wrapped in tinsel is still garbage," Dr. Spencer intoned, his Southern drawl intensifying with his clear-cut disdain. "And what did Osler know anyway? He was a young pup pathologist from the Canadian prairies. He learned his bedside manner on cadavers."

—⋙—

Patients, who are on the receiving end of what students are learning from teachers like Frank Spencer—or what they are not learning—have the most at stake here. It's not surprising that surveys find that patients are more satisfied with empathic doctors, but whether empathy affects patients' actual physical health is a more tenuous etiologic stretch.

Studying hard outcomes of physician empathy on patients' health is a new field, but the preliminary outcomes are intriguing. One study showed that the patients of doctors with higher empathy scores have better control of their cholesterol and blood sugar.[12] Medication compliance appears to be increased for patients with more empathic doctors.[13] Oncology patients may experience better quality of life and less depression with empathic practitioners.[14] Even the basic common cold could possibly be influenced. The colds of patients with more empathic doctors were less severe and ended sooner.[15]

In one of the largest studies of its type, more than 20,000 diabetic patients of 242 doctors were analyzed for the severest swings of glucose—the type of hyper- and hypoglycemia that leads to hospitalization and coma. The doctors all took the JSE empathy test and were divided into groups with high, moderate, or low scores. The rate of severe diabetes complications in patients of high-empathy doctors was 40 percent lower than that of patients with low-empathy doctors.[16] This is comparable to the benefits seen with the most intensive medical therapy for diabetes, except that those treatments also cause significant side effects. (So far, there haven't been any documented "adverse outcomes" in patients treated by highly empathic doctors.)

It's not clear whether outcomes change because the doctor is a more astute listener and picks up keys to illness that other doctors miss or because the patients feel more secure and more able to do what they need to do in order to heal themselves. These specific etiologies will be difficult to parse, but it may not be necessary to be reductionist about it.

Sir William Osler was an internist in addition to being a pathologist, and so he had plenty of live patients as well as dead ones. He is reputed to have said (and he may have been restating Hippocrates here): "It is much more important to know what sort of a patient has a disease than what sort of a disease a patient has." To me, this is an excellent working definition of empathy.

James Easton—the elderly patient with the horrific ulcers that required both legs to be amputated—was one of the hardest patients to take care of. The medical care per se was actually straightforward—antibiotics and dressing changes. But just being in his room, witnessing his body, was unsettling to everyone, especially the resident on our team. I would see her shaking her head, muttering softly to herself, "Those ulcers are incompatible with life. I can't understand how he is still alive." The decision to undertake amputation—a formidable surgery, given his weakened medical condition—was an ethical quandary. His quality of life seemed to be nil, seemingly worse than a comatose patient because of how little actual body was left.

Then one day, shortly after Mr. Easton was admitted, the resident came running toward me in the doctors' station, almost breathless. "Mr. Easton's family is here," she exclaimed. Family? Mr. Easton had family?

Somehow, we hadn't imagined that someone like him had a family. He had seemed so unmoored physically and mentally that we assumed he was unmoored socially too. It was as though his drastic physical appearance made him seem not human in every respect.

Of course, none of this had been processed consciously, and we certainly didn't stand on rounds discussing how unhuman Mr. Easton looked. But in retrospect, I can see that this was how we were feeling. We were so deeply unsettled by Mr. Easton's body, by seeing someone whose physical condition appeared incompatible with life, that we reacted by shutting him out of our moral vision.

But the arrival of his wife changed that in an instant. A stout, no-nonsense woman wearing a Sunday-best green suit with matching green heels and flowered hat, she was as vivid as her husband was faint. She bustled into the room with an armload of daisies, rearranged the chairs and nightstand, and pinned a panoply of prayer cards on his wall.

For the resident in particular, Mrs. Easton's arrival lifted an enormous burden. It was clear that she'd been agonizing over the difficulty in relating to her patient. But now there was a connection. The phrase *incompatible with life* never came up again.

Mrs. Easton told us how a series of strokes had debilitated her husband, confining him to bed, and how his severe diabetes and old heroin habits had destroyed his ability to heal, allowing infections and ulcers to always remain several steps ahead of his doctors. She had moved him from nursing home to nursing home, but the ulcers kept gouging deeper into his limbs. "He used to be a preacher," she told us. "But now he only preaches inside his head. You can tell when he's preaching, because his eyes light up in that special way."

It was like we'd been looking into an unfocused microscope, seeing only murky smudges, and Mrs. Easton had yanked the dial from our blundering fingers and wrenched the image into focus. With the arrival of his wife, Mr. Easton suddenly appeared as a human being—one with a life story, with a tapestry of connections, with dimensions beyond the current diminished physical state he was in. We were startled to see what sort of person had this disease, rather than what sort of disease this person had.

You could argue that we should have been able to see Mr. Easton's humanity even without his wife, and you would be right; we should have. But we couldn't. Our fears, anxieties, prejudices, and short-sightedness got the better of us. Luckily for us—and for our future patients—Mrs. Easton graced the scene.

Julia, part two

Eight years had elapsed between the day we gave Julia her death sentence and that incongruously gorgeous autumn day that she tumbled off the Starling curve. Between those hellish bookends, her overall health was surprisingly excellent. Though her heart was insidiously worsening, every other organ, muscle, and sinew in her body was young and robust. Her cardiology team took advantage of this and worked aggressively to titrate an armada of medications that kept her CHF symptoms at bay. Julia was meticulous about her panoply of pills, keeping track of changing doses, medications that were added, medications that were discontinued, frequent medical appointments, and never-ending blood tests required for fine-tuning the precarious pharmaceutical equilibrium—all while speaking nary a word of English. It wasn't easy, but Julia possessed a quiet tenacity, motivated largely by the two children for whose sake she desperately wanted to live.

During those eight years, we had frequent medical visits together to keep tabs on her ever-changing cardiac regimen. Julia looked perfectly healthy. And she felt healthy too. She climbed the three flights of stairs to her apartment, cared for her children, negotiated life. If she had been sixty-five years old with hypertension, diabetes, obesity, and a handful of heart attacks under her belt, she would have been dead already. But the combination of youth, health, good medical care, and sheer luck had Julia disproving the textbooks.

To look at her, you wouldn't know.

But I did know. And she knew. And so our medical visits felt surreal. My eyes saw a healthy young mother, but inside I knew the fragility of her existence. Every time I listened to the tenuous thrum of her heart, my own heart clenched up. Each time we said good-bye, I feared it could be our last.

I knew that when the moment came, her heart's relentless downward spiral would overcome every scrap of health in the rest of her body, every determined cardiologist, every prayer her family and friends dutifully offered in church. There would be nothing to do. The ephemeral image of a heart transplant would taunt us like a cruel specter as we watched her succumb to a brutal death. All because of her immigration status.

During those eight years, though, much transpired in both of our lives. Her American-born daughter Lucita entered kindergarten. My younger daughter, Ariel, was born during my sabbatical in Costa Rica. Julia and I shared stories of complicated citizenships for our daughters, the challenges of keeping up Spanish and English.

Julia's older son, Vasco, had been left behind in Guatemala with his grandmother. Julia and her husband saved their money, and when Vasco was eight, they finally had the $4,500 it cost to bring him across the border. But it didn't go well. Vasco tripped while sprinting through the rugged desert, losing his shoe. Immigration officials descended upon them. The coyotes abandoned the boy, dashing off for their own safety. Learning-disabled after severe meningitis as an infant, Vasco was unable to remember the fake name he was supposed to use. He ended up in custody for months in Texas before the paperwork could be completed and Julia's brother could make the trip there to claim him. Vasco was now reunited with his parents, though he was having trouble in school because of behavioral issues related to his disability.

All those years, I wrestled with my emotions during my visits with Julia. She preferred not to talk about the big picture, so I followed her lead and left it out of our conversations. Frankly, that made it easier for me. I could dwell within my own denial, focusing simply on the minor issues of the day. But I felt guilty about this. I felt as though Julia and I were colluding in a grand scheme to pretend that the ultimate day would never arrive. I knew this pseudo-health was a mirage, but I so desperately wanted it to be true that I allowed myself to indulge.

That fall morning was the end of my denial. When I walked into the hospital, still vitalized from the autumn fragrance, I could tell immediately from Julia's pale, wan look that she wasn't okay. When she told me that the slightest movement of her body felt like she was "swimming through mud," I knew that we were in trouble. I paged her cardiologist and we admitted her straight to the ICU. There was a slight chance that this could be something reversible—an infection, a medication issue, a slight hiccup in her equilibrium—and I clung to that hope.

Unfortunately, it was none of those. It was just the progression of her disease. While she was being treated with aggressive medications to try to relieve the pressure on her heart, I put my own pressure on the cardiologist. "Is there any way," I begged him, "that she could get on the transplant list?"

I'd called the organ donation organization myself and learned that 1 percent of organs went to foreigners, though no one could tell me if these were undocumented immigrants, foreign royalty, or tourists. But at least there was a chance, however slim.

The cardiology fellow had explained to me that it wasn't just the issue of getting the actual transplant but also the challenge of the ongoing complex immunosuppressive medications. Without insurance, these medications ran $10,000 per year. A transplant candidate needed insurance or money, not to mention a stable social network to support her through the entire daunting process.

I'd been working on my book *Medicine in Translation* at the time and had written the story of our difficulty in giving Julia her diagnosis. Now, with a heavy heart, I added in Julia's latest setback and my conversation with the cardiologist. He didn't seem hopeful, but he was willing to try.

"I did my residency at Columbia," the cardiology fellow said. "I know the transplant people there and I'll present her case. Let's see if we can get them to take her."

"What happens if they don't?" I asked.

"We'll talk to the folks at Mount Sinai. They have a smaller program, but they're worth a shot."

"What happens if they don't take her?"

"Well, we'll try at Montefiore."

"And if that doesn't work?"

He was silent.[1]

CHAPTER 3

Scared Witless

The stat cardiac-arrest page came through on my beeper at exactly the same moment as the hospital-wide PA system announced, "Code 411, cardiac arrest, MICU." The operator chanted the mantra over and over with studied deliberativeness, as though there were even a snowball's chance in hell that I hadn't heard it. The repetitive droning of her voice echoing throughout the twenty-three floors of the hospital and the persistent buzzing of the beeper at my waist were like rising tides of terror pressing in on both sides of me.

This was it—the first code I was in charge of.

After two years of racing to codes as a first- and second-year resident, buoyed by the excitement of dramatic action, thrilled to be part of a team, grateful to be assigned one of the many minute tasks required to save a life, secure in the knowledge that the medical consult would be directing the show—now suddenly, the code was mine. I was the medical consult. I was the one to call the shots, to direct the care, to assign the jobs, to make the decisions.

I had been on the medical-consult service for less than a week. I'd been privately counting on thirty days elapsing with every last coronary artery in the hospital capaciously wide open, every lung alveolus buoyant with oxygen, every blood clot obediently self-dissolving, but this strategy was evidently not working as I'd hoped. Here it was: my first code.

Shit!

I slapped my hands against the overloaded pockets of my white coat to keep the tools and cards and pocket guides from spilling out while I raced to the medical intensive care unit. I burst into the MICU breathless, throat parched to Saharan levels, pulse pounding powerfully enough to detonate the collar of my shirt, and glanced wildly about the unit.

There was the crowd, huddled around bed 5. I loped over and pressed through the bodies, angling toward the head of the bed. "I'm med consult," I announced, gamely smoothing out the jitteriness in my voice.

And then my brain splintered into complete and utter blackness.

A resident began feeding me the facts—seventy-two-year-old guy, diabetes, coronary disease, stroke last year, admitted with pneumonia, developed allergic reaction to his antibiotics, subsequent renal insufficiency, transferred to the MICU three days ago for congestive heart failure, spiked a fever last night, a bit delirious but still talking, now unresponsive, BP 70 over palp, thready pulse.

Or something like that. The truth was, I couldn't have told you the details twenty seconds after he finished relaying them to me, much less twenty years later. Everything he said sloshed into the primordial neuronal soup that was now the condition of my gray matter.

Say something, I implored myself. *Anything.* "Chest compressions," I forced out. "Keep bagging the oxygen. Get a line in. EKG."

Any idiot knows the basics for keeping someone alive! But what next? My brain remained jammed up with panic. I couldn't seem to remember a damn thing from those ACLS training courses. All the protocols had seemed so logical then, so ridiculously simple on those ever-forgiving mannequins.

But now there was someone real, someone alive—though perhaps not for much longer with me at the helm—and I couldn't unknot a single protocol.

Did you shock first or give epinephrine first? Or was epi only for the asystole algorithm? Should I be following the pulseless electrical activity algorithm? Or the pulseless ventricular tachycardia algorithm?

Someone pressed an EKG into my hand. The presence of something actual in my hands brought a brief mollifying reprieve of emotion. These would be my tablets handed down from the Mount; the talismanic markings would allow me to divine the answer and jump-start my fear-stricken brain.

I stared at the electrocardiogram. And stared. And stared. I squinted at the zigs and the zags, but they seemed to melt into a Sanskrit-like jumble. *Think*, I demanded. *Think!* All those exhortations from my teachers about approaching the EKG methodically, about systematically examining the rhythm, the rate, the axis, the P waves, the QRS complexes, the T waves—these lessons evaporated in the cold shudder of reality.

Think, I screamed to myself.

Okay, the T waves. Maybe they looked a little peaked. Peaked T waves were indicative of elevated potassium levels, except when they weren't. And except when they looked peaked but weren't actually peaked.

They did look sort of peaked, I thought to myself, but maybe they were just hyperacute T waves, or maybe they were enlarged from early repolarization. Or maybe they were just big. I was too terrified to trust myself on anything. I could order the treatment for hyper-kalemia—if those peaked T waves were real—but I was too scared that I might be wrong. What if I injected intravenous calcium for hy-perkalemia that wasn't actually there, then really fucked things up?

"Who's in charge here, anyway?" barked a new voice. My body seized up tighter, if that was even possible. A cardiology fellow blus-tered his way into the crowd, clearly seeing the mess for what it was. I looked up and made a vague indication that I was running the code.

There was an embarrassing moment as the fellow and I instantly recognized each other—Mitchell had been in my medical-school class. We'd spent the first two years of school together, even traveled in the same circle of friends. But because of the years I'd taken to do my PhD, he'd completed his training before me and was now a senior cardiology fellow while I was a third-year medical resident.

It was evident that if he hadn't known me from med-school days he would have dressed down the medical consult for not running the code more aggressively. He bit back his comment, sidled over to me, and leaned in to look at the EKG. "Peaked T waves, hyperkalemia," he announced clearly, though not derisively—an act of humanity that allowed me a modicum of dignity. "Let's get some calcium," he said, "an amp of bicarb, D50 and insulin."

The patient did all right in the end, or at least survived the code, which was pretty much what we considered success in the MICU. I slunk off after the patient stabilized, hoping to disappear myself in the sea of white coats shuffling off to conference or rounds or the ER. I was furious at myself for getting so paralyzed by fear that I could barely run the code. What had happened to all my training? All the codes I'd participated in? All the lectures and books I'd been learning from?

What made me the angriest at myself, though, was that I'd actually gotten it right. It *was* hyperkalemia. The T waves absolutely had been peaked. I could have called it on the spot and been the model of a take-charge resident, as a medical consult running a code is supposed to be. But I couldn't get beyond my gripping fear—of the situation, of getting it wrong, of killing the patient, of looking like an idiot.

—⁓—

The amygdala is ground zero for the processing of fear in human beings.[1] I remember the first time I laid eyes on an actual amygdala, after slicing through a brain with a repurposed kitchen knife in neuroanatomy class. *That's it?* I thought. That nickel-size splotch tucked below the temporal lobes was the seat of my fears? It was monumentally underwhelming and even lacked the poetic almond shape that its Latin name connotes.

The amygdala acts as the ringleader of the limbic system—the emotional guts of our brain. Weaving together the hippocampus, thalamus, amygdala, and some ancient parts of the cerebral cortex, the limbic system calibrates the nitty-gritty of who we are—our fears, our attractions, our memories, not to mention the cornerstone imperatives of food, sex, and anger. If psychoanalysis had a neuroanatomical substrate, it would be the limbic system. And if it wanted a laser-like focus, especially when it comes to fear, it would train its sights on the amygdala.

I read of a patient with a rare condition that damaged the amygdala on both sides of her brain. Though her other emotions appeared normal, she neither felt nor expressed fear. Researchers did what they could to frighten her—brought in live snakes, set spiders loose, showed scary movies.[2] They even took her on a haunted-house tour. She didn't so much as flinch. It wasn't that she had nerves of steel; she simply did not experience fear.

As a medical student and intern, I longed to be her. I desperately desired an emotional shield that would block out the paralyzing fear that seemed to track my every step. If I could only corral my amygdala and limbic system, being a doctor would be effortless.

Fear is a primal emotion in medicine. Every doctor can tell you of times when she or he was terrified; most can list more episodes than you might wish to hear. This fear of making a mistake and causing harm never goes away, even with decades of experience. It may be most palpable and expressible in neophyte students and interns, but that is merely the first link in a chain that wends its way throughout the life of a doctor. It may be sublimated at times, it may wax and wane, but the fear of harming your patients never departs; it is inextricably linked to the practice of medicine.

I sometimes compare career notes with friends who are in the business world, and I've asked what their worst fear is. It's usually something along the lines of making a financial blunder, screwing up a major project, having an investment fall apart, losing a job, disappointing the boss or family, losing money. I have to restrain myself from saying, *That's it? That's all you are afraid of?*

That, of course, is the basic fear in medicine, that we will kill someone, or cause palpable bodily harm. I vividly remember my first reading of Ernest Becker's classic existential treatise *The Denial of Death*.[3] Becker posited that humans are terrified of their own mortality, and that every action we take, on an individual or societal level, is directed (usually unconsciously) by the necessary denial of imminent death.

This precisely captured my fear as a doctor-in-training, except that the fear was entirely conscious. I was terrified of causing death, and every action I took was an obeisance to that fear. Medical students, for all of their competence and competitiveness, are a pretty fearful bunch, more so than the general population and even more than their age-matched peers pursuing other professions.[4] Some of this is not surprising. You really *should* possess some fear as you begin to jab sharp objects into other people's bodies, prescribe potentially lethal medicines, or initiate treatments that put lives at risk. Any medical student without fear is a cavalier cowboy better suited to a desk job.

But the fears can easily spiral out of control and overwhelm students and interns. If this happened only rarely, to only those few who entered the medical field with their own preexisting mental-health conditions, that would be one thing. But the truth is that the fear overwhelms even the most psychologically sound and well-adjusted trainee. At some point it happens to nearly every single person who travels through the medical training process. If you don't believe me, just ask any doctor you know.

—⁓—

Curtis Climer has traveled extensively, but at heart he is a rooted person. He practices medicine in the very same rural Oregon hospital in which he was born. His family has lived in Oregon since the early 1800s. His grandmother was one of ten siblings, but in the vast extended family that descended from her, there was only one other cousin beside Curtis who even attended college. Curtis is the first physician in the family.

Medical school was a shock for him. Coming from a tiny college, where asking questions in class was encouraged and quirky humor was comfortably tolerated, Curtis didn't blend in with the conservative students from big universities. Nobody laughed at his jokes. They rolled their eyes derisively every time he raised his hand in class, and he was awarded the prize for Most Ridiculous Question of the Year at the school's annual awards ceremony. The bushy lumberjack beard didn't help.

But by the second year, things improved. Spending the summer in the fresh air at a summer camp teaching gymnastics (he'd been a gymnast all through college) gave a lift to his spirits. When he re-entered the lecture halls with a new attitude and a new clean-shaven look, many of his classmates didn't even know who he was. Gradually he came to know them, and they turned out not to be so awful. The feeling was mutual. "You know, I thought you were so weird," one of his classmates said in the backhanded-compliment style of a twenty-something, "but you're actually pretty ordinary."

When internship arrived, Curtis flourished. He loved the specificity of clinical medicine. In the classroom, he'd had to memorize reams of diseases, all of which had equal emphasis. But on the wards, a patient's symptoms narrowed this list, made certain diseases more likely, and often pointed to one specific disease, something you could actually hang your hat on, something you could focus on treating. The day-to-day work, however, was exhausting and he never seemed to be able to catch up on sleep. The endless paging and constant multitasking made him feel like a battery that was always draining, never recharging.

That January morning was like all others, the start of another thirty-six-hour call day—ten sick patients on his hands, plus four new admissions already waiting for him. It was the dark days of winter, and Curtis couldn't remember the last time he'd seen an actual ray of sunshine. Before he'd even had his first yawn of the morning, a gastric ulcer in one of his patients chose that moment to begin hemorrhaging. Curtis dropped everything and sprinted down the hall, his mind spinning through his mental list—check vitals, two large-bore IVs, fluids wide open, stat hematocrit, call blood bank for two units of blood on standby, rectal exam to see if there was blood in the stool, nasogastric tube to lavage stomach, page GI if patient crashing.

While he was stabilizing the GI bleeder, at the other end of the ward a blood clot was casually flicked out of the heart of another of Curtis's patients. Shortly thereafter, the patient couldn't move the left side of his body. Curtis shifted gears and flew to stanch that fire, his brain now flipping to the protocol for acute stroke—check vitals, quick neuro exam, stat head CT, page neuro. The four new admissions were still waiting in the emergency room, of course. And there was still the daily litany of morning report, attending rounds, noon conference. It really wasn't different than any other day.

The day wore on into evening. The calls from nurses for various emergencies large and small continued unabated. By nightfall, the calls shifted to tasks that his colleagues had neglected to do before they'd left—medication renewals, IV replacements, sundry forms and orders. At 10:30 that night, Curtis remembers getting annoyed at his compatriots for not being more assiduous at clearing up their scut lists.

He was sitting at a desk on Unit 4C writing a progress note in a chart when his pager went off for the umpteenth time. He dialed the phone automatically, still penning his note, and a nurse requested an order for Tylenol. A Tylenol order for an intern requires even less thought than flicking on a light switch. It's a task that barely registers on the horizon of consciousness.

But at this moment, Curtis suddenly had no idea what to say. He couldn't remember the first thing about Tylenol—how much, how often. "Somewhere inside of me," he recalls, "I could feel myself falling backward off a cliff. I was in free fall and could actually feel the wind blowing by me. I could see the edge of the cliff growing smaller as I fell deeper and deeper into some ill-defined chasm. And I had no idea where bottom was."

He stammered incomprehensibly on the phone. The nonplussed nurse prompted him, feeding him the details of 650 mg PO, q4H, prn, and he mumbled his assent as tears began to fill his eyes. He hung up the phone and simply sat there, stunned, weeping.

"I had no idea what had happened," he says now. "All I knew was that it felt like I could not make another decision." When his pager went off again, it was for a simple sleeping medication, one that he had prescribed dozens of times in the past month. But he couldn't dredge up any information about it. He stumbled through the conversation somehow, then he called his resident, Mike.

"What do you need?" Mike asked briskly. A good resident was always on the prowl to lift an item or two off his intern's scut list.

"I'm not sure, Mike," Curtis said hesitantly. "Something is wrong."

"What's the matter?" Mike asked, his voice beginning to register the gravity of the situation.

"I . . . I don't know," Curtis replied, and the tears began to flow again.

"Stay where you are," Mike said. "I'll be right over. *Don't move.*"

Curtis hunched over his shoulders and sat in the doctors' station, crying, waiting, praying that his pager would not go off. Mike arrived at 4C promptly and didn't seem fazed by a sobbing intern. He seemed to know what was happening.

"Give me your scut list," he said calmly to Curtis. "I'll take care of this. You get over to the call room and get as much sleep as you can." Curtis raised himself shakily to his feet. His physical body seemed to work, but everything inside had shut down.

"Tomorrow morning," Mike ordered, "skip any work or meetings that are not absolutely critical. By whatever means possible, you need to be out of the hospital by noon. I'll pick up whatever is left over to do."

Curtis shuffled off to the call room, only vaguely able to process the compassion of his resident. The beds were rumpled and old; the sheets probably hadn't been changed from the last four interns, but he didn't care. He dropped off into a dense and dreamless sleep. When he awoke, he was still standing on the cliff, but now he was four feet inland from the edge. Four feet of safety but still four feet from the chasm. He could easily topple over again.

He worked cautiously through his morning tasks, not sure if the oddness inside him was visible to the outside world. But just after attending rounds, Kathryn, the other intern on the team, leaned over and said, "Curtis, what's happening to you?"

Curtis explained to her about the Tylenol and the cliff and the black, bottomless abyss. She listened carefully, and then very softly she said, "That's your first time, right?"

He stared back at her, too amazed to speak.

"For most of us," she continued, "it's already happened several times. For some it started within the first month of internship."

Curtis was stunned. One experience like this was terrifying; he could not imagine going through it repeatedly. With Mike's help, he managed to escape the hospital by noon. Once home, he took a steaming bath and then crashed on his bed, not stirring for the next seventeen hours. When he awoke the next day he was twenty feet back from the cliff edge. He felt better, more like his regular self. He probably would not fall off from that twenty-foot distance, but he knew now that he could, and that disquieting knowledge could not be unlearned.

—⁓—

Curtis experienced an acute stress reaction, a psychological term that encompasses a spectrum of responses. The common thread is an intense reaction to a shocking or traumatic event. The sympathetic nervous system shifts into overdrive, and tides of hormones and neuronal firings can alter the state of being, sometimes profoundly. Gravely injured patients can be in a state of shock so profound that they sense no pain whatsoever.

Different people exhibit different reactions to the same stressor— sometimes diametric opposites. Witnessing a person keel over unconscious can induce such overwhelming panic and anxiety in a bystander that he or she freezes, unable to do anything. For the next person over, this stressor can sharpen their focus and nerve, allowing them to jump in and begin CPR.

What Curtis experienced is termed a dissociative reaction. He felt utterly removed from himself, wicked away from the events around him. There is a sense of the surreal, as the real world waxes and wanes.

Anecdotally, many doctors and nurses will tell you about their "moments," as they are often called, that moment when the medical world overwhelmed them and they were unable to function for some period. But there is little research in the field. What has been published shows that for health professionals, acute stress worsens performance on tasks that require divided attention—that is, tasks that require integrating information from various sources.[5] In contrast, concrete tasks that require selective attention—placing an IV, for example—may be improved by a modest amount of stress.

But complex tasks requiring attention to disparate things suffer notably under stress conditions. Multitasking and juggling is the daily bread of medicine—treating a patient who has stomach pain but also a rash and also missed three days of medications; taking a phone call from an anxious family member or irate insurance company while documenting the details of a physical exam; reacting to a dangerously low sodium level but remembering that the treatment is different depending on the patient's overall fluid status while also remembering to check whether the low sodium is merely an artifact related to concomitant hyperglycemia.

Curtis's acute stress reaction was not uncommon, as his fellow intern noted. For him, it was a reaction to the composite of his situation. The Tylenol request was simply the trigger that nudged him over the edge, almost literally. His reaction—and the signal that something needed to be done—was loud and clear, and luckily Curtis had a resident who recognized the situation immediately. Very often, however, these signs are missed.

Some medical schools and residency programs are taking note of the fact that fear, stress, and feelings of being overwhelmed are nearly universal in their trainees, and are beginning to take steps to address this. This is crucial, because research from the field of psychology suggests that people who are fearful are more pessimistic in their outlook and may overestimate the risk of bad outcome.[6] As a result, their choices of action may lean toward the risk-averse.

As I stood in front of my first coding patient, I "chose" what seemed to be the most risk-averse action—doing nothing—even though it turned out that I'd made the correct diagnosis of elevated potassium. At that moment, doing nothing seemed the least risky path, but it wasn't. If the cardiology fellow hadn't come along in time, my patient would have died promptly from a hyperkalemic cardiac arrest.

What exactly is going on? Why does overwhelming anxiety so brutally impair our decision-making? The amygdala and the limbic system figure prominently here,[7] as a welter of emotions distracts us, and we misread important cues. There is a tendency to overemphasize the unimportant issues while downgrading the important ones. I can remember the swell of stimuli—people shouting, machines beeping, equipment flying—and how it seemed to cave in on my thought process, making it impossible to concentrate on the critical tasks at hand.

Some residency programs offer stress-management workshops, support groups and mindfulness meditation.[8] Other suggestions for reducing stress range from identifying and treating trainees who exhibit "at-risk" behavior to increasing "interdisciplinary teamwork" to rejiggering call schedules to chewing gum[9] (yes, gum does seem to reduce stress, at least in undergrads). But in the end, most residents are simply too busy to incorporate yet another thing, no matter how beneficial, into their day,[10] or maybe it's just too difficult for doctors to practice medicine and chew gum at the same time.

A surgery residency in Greece taught half of its residents simple stress-reduction techniques, such as muscle relaxation and deep breathing, over the course of two months. Compared to their colleagues who didn't undergo this training, these surgical residents experienced a significant decrease in their stress levels and a concomitant increase in their decision-making abilities.[11]

Though these programs seek to reduce stress—in the global sense of all things awful about medical training—none really focuses on the fear, the panic really, that grips us during various points in our careers. There are many who argue that doctors should never lose the fear of doing harm, that it is a healthy existential fear that maintains a necessary awe and humility in a field where lives are indeed at stake. But for those in the profession, we need to be alert for when we or our colleagues become overwhelmed by this fear; our patients' lives are at stake.

Over the years of practice, as I gained confidence, I found that my overriding fear receded in intensity, though it never completely vanished. Studies have corroborated that stress generally decreases as one moves along in training.[12] My fear became, perhaps more in parallel with Ernest Becker's theory, an unconscious, or maybe semiconscious, modulator of my actions. The moments of utter panic were fewer, but the fear was never absent.

—⚏—

Hao Zhong was a thirty-two-year-old man who had swallowed a bottle of pills and then followed this by slitting his wrists with a carving knife. "He's stable," my resident told me—I was the attending in charge of the ward for that month—"but his family wants him transferred to Mount Sinai."

This is a frequent occurrence with upper-middle-class patients who accidentally end up in a public hospital. The ambulance brings them to the closest facility that can handle the particular emergency. (For Mr. Zhong, with his dramatic suicide attempt, that facility was, of course, Bellevue Hospital.) Then, when they realize where they are, they start clamoring—sometimes demanding—a transfer to a private hospital.

When they become aware that they will have to pay out of pocket for the transfer, however, many change their minds and settle in. More often than not, they find themselves pleasantly surprised by the clean, spacious hospital and doctors quite similar to their private physicians. However, I never press anyone to stay at Bellevue (unless his medical condition would make leaving unsafe). My feeling is that if someone prefers to be at a private hospital and is able to make the arrangements, then he should go where he is most comfortable.

Mr. Zhong didn't care one way or another, but his family wanted him uptown in the swankier setting that Mount Sinai offered. The resident told me that the arrangements were in progress. Psych had seen the patient in the ER but wanted him monitored on the medical ward because of the pills he'd swallowed. I called hospital administration, because I always forget the precise details of interhospital transfer. "If they want to arrange an ambulance and can pay for it, they are free to go," an administrator told me. "But it's not *our* responsibility to take care of the arrangements. It's the family's."

I was listening with only half an ear. I had started on the wards just the day before and was supervising two teams of residents, each with eighteen to twenty patients. The day wasn't more than half over, but I was already behind the eight ball, still trying to get a handle on the old patients while a steady stream of new admissions was coming in, including Mr. Zhong.

I scanned my spreadsheet with thirty-nine typed names, plus several more handwritten at the bottom, each scribbled in as a new admission arrived. Starting on the wards was always harrowing. It seemed impossible to familiarize myself with every patient, but I had to be sure that I leafed through every chart and at least stopped in at every patient's room for a brief visit, since I was ultimately responsible for every single patient on our ward. Even that minimal amount of attention, though, took hours. I worried incessantly that something would slip under the radar.

I plowed my way through 16-West, checking in with each patient on my list to be sure everything was okay, at least for the moment. I told myself that I would review each case in depth on the following day. Though tomorrow the other team under my supervision would be admitting, so there would be another influx of new patients. The residents and interns were scurrying about with today's new admissions, while I scurried about getting familiar with the old patients. Whenever our paths crossed, we would confer briefly over the latest lab results, pending X-rays, or minor crises that arose. It wasn't humanly possible for me to check every lab on every patient; I relied on my residents.

Mr. Zhong was resting comfortably in his bed when I popped into his room. He was wearing a white undershirt and old sweatpants, but his hyper-trendy European eyeglasses gave away his socioeconomic status. As did his high-end laptop, upon which he was typing furiously. "IPO's in a few days," he said, by way of explanation. "Still ironing out kinks in the security codes."

When I peeled back the bandages on his wrists, I could see that the cuts he'd made were superficial. They didn't even require stitches, only surgical adhesive strips. "I was pretty stupid, eh?" he said, pursing his lips in a self-deprecatory manner.

"Well," I said, leaning against the wall near his bed since the visitors' chair had apparently been requisitioned elsewhere, "it depends on how you look at it. You certainly sent a clear message to your family and to your doctors that something serious is going on in your life."

"It's not like I want to die or anything—" he replied, then cut himself off midsentence. "That's sounds pretty ridiculous, doesn't it? I mean, here I am sitting in Bellevue, for God's sake." He gave an eye roll but also smiled wryly. "I mean, how stupid can I get? Just because at three in the morning I couldn't think of a better way to cut the stress. And now my partner's gonna kick my butt if I don't get the last bug out of the system. Maybe I ought to slit the wrists of my computer." He shot an exaggerated glare at the laptop.

Because of the overdose, the ER had lavaged his stomach and administered a dose of charcoal to absorb whatever the lavage might have missed. This apparently worked, because his body seemed to have suffered few ill effects. His labs and EKG were normal. Mr. Zhong said he was feeling fine and was mostly sheepish about his suicide attempt. "I gotta go back to my old shrink—you don't need to tell me that." But of course I did tell him that, and we discussed the importance of ongoing treatment.

When I pressed him about further thoughts of suicide or concrete plans, he shook his head. "If I kill myself and botch the IPO, my partner will kill me." He stopped and his face took on a mock-perplexed look. "No, wait, that won't work, will it."

Onward through the ward I soldiered. Mrs. Everett's fever was down. Mr. Liang was getting his chemo. Mr. Chowdury was waiting to be called down for his stress test. Mrs. Jimenez had been accepted by a nursing home, but the bed wasn't ready yet. Mr. Selwin was in the GI suite getting his endoscopy. Ms. Soto's bone scan hadn't been read yet. Mr. Hastings would be discharged after ophthalmology saw him. Mr. Sabatini was refusing an IV. Mrs. Abaza had been at dialysis since 8:00 a.m. Mr. Riyad needed only two more days of antibiotics. Cardiology would be taking Mr. Vladic to the cath suite any minute now.

By late afternoon I'd gotten through most of my list, though the new admissions continued to pile up. The stable ones—pyelonephritis and noncardiac chest pain—I'd put off till later. The GI bleeder I checked on right away.

The only thing that made it possible for an attending to be in charge of forty patients was that the interns and residents were actually the primary doctors for the patients and did the direct work. I functioned more as the supervisor and consultant to my two house-staff teams. I of course had to check on every patient myself, but they did the grunt work.

The sun was edging down into the East River as I sank into one of the seen-better-days office chairs in the doctors' station with six charts open in front of me, consulting my patient list and making notes. The resident popped in. "The ambulance is here to transfer Mr. Zhong to Sinai."

I looked up and saw medics wearing sporty blue parkas standing with a stretcher in front of the nurses' station. "All his labs okay?" I asked the resident.

"Yep," he said. "It's been twenty-four hours since ingestion now, and no change."

"Seen by psych?"

"Evaluated in the ER."

"Someone's called his private psychiatrist?"

"Yep."

"There's an accepting doctor at Mount Sinai?"

"Yep."

"Family took care of papers, transfer issues, ambulance?"

"Yep."

"Okay," I said. "Wish him well. Did Sanders get the head CT yet?"

"Med students are wheeling her down now. I'll call you when the results are back." The resident was already out the door with three scut lists in his hand.

I watched Mr. Zhong climb onto the stretcher, surrounded by his family. When he saw me through the window he pointed to the laptop under his arm and made a scissors-snipping motion at it. I couldn't help but smile. The medics tucked the sheets around him and then buckled the orange safety belts that prevented the patient from slipping off while the stretcher was in motion. Papers were signed, and he was off. I waved and then turned back to my charts; the chair creaked its annoyance at my movements.

Mr. Lambert had spiked a new fever. Ms. Hestina needed an ENT consultation, but that could wait until tomorrow. The surgeons wanted medical clearance in order to take Mr. Kinsawa to the OR, so we'd need to take care of that now. That antibiotic for Mr. Demir was nonformulary, so needed a special approval form. Mrs. Jennings was refusing her meds.

The phone rang, and I answered while scanning my list. It was the hospital administrator I'd spoken to earlier. "That patient of yours who wanted to go to Mount Sinai," he said. "I was just looking at his record and I see that he was admitted for a suicide attempt. Did psych clear him?"

"They saw him in the ER," I replied, pulling over a nonformulary medication form and filling in Mr. Demir's details.

"Yes, but that was just the emergency consultation in the ER. Did the regular psych team evaluate him once he was up on 16-West?"

A sudden iron tension burrowed in my spine. "On 16-West?" I stammered, my mind now beginning to shift gears. "Umm, I know they saw him in the ER, but I don't know if they were here on the ward. We were told the patient was cleared in the ER." I shoved the form away and started scrambling through the charts on my desk to see if Mr. Zhong's was there, which of course it wasn't.

"Dr. Ofri." The administrator's tone turned stern. "You sent a potentially suicidal patient out of the hospital?"

"He went in an ambulance, with medics." I could hear my voice trying to shore up the situation with whatever hard facts I had at hand.

"He went in the care of his family in a private ambulance. They could take him anywhere they want. They could take him home. They could leave him on the street." The administrator continued to lecture me, but my nerves were already jangling with anxiety and it was difficult to focus. "If something happens to him, if he attempts suicide again, we are entirely responsible! You can't let a patient like this out of the hospital."

I raced to the nurses' station, pulled out Mr. Zhong's chart from the discharge bin, and began flipping madly through the pages. I finally found the original ER sheet and scanned through twenty-four hours of handwritten notes. Scrawled at the bottom was the psych note: *Patient with strong supports and family network. Not currently voicing interest in repeat suicide attempt, but nevertheless remains at risk. Would keep on 1:1 observation until re-evaluated by regular psych consult team.*

The regular psych consult team! How could we have missed that? Now we had gone and discharged a patient whose last psych evaluation said to keep on 1:1 observation for suicide precaution. If anything happened to Mr. Zhong . . . I could hardly bring myself to think it. I dropped the chart on the desk and haltingly drew both hands to my mouth as the gravity of what I might have done began to sink in. What if my oversight caused the death of this young man? And, of course, on the legal side of things, I wouldn't have so much as a toothpick to stand on.

Back in the doctors' station I threw myself into the chair, ignoring the angry hissing of the cushion. I grabbed the phone and snapped at the operator for Mount Sinai's phone number. I had visions of Mr. Zhong bolting out of the ambulance and streaking down Third Avenue, disappearing into the night, swallowed up by the anonymous city. Would he fling himself on the subway tracks? Dodge in front of a careening taxi? Clean out the Tylenol shelf at CVS and swallow his way to fulminant liver failure?

I wended through layers of phone tree at Mount Sinai, trying to ascertain whether Hao Zhong had arrived there. I kept getting low-level administrators who curtly declined my request for information, citing HIPAA privacy regulations. I slammed the phone down and gritted my teeth. How could I have been so stupid!

I saw my resident walking briskly down the hall with the rest of the team. They all clutched charts and scut lists and were talking and writing as they walked. I could hardly blame them for this mess.

Too much was happening at once. They'd gotten a verbal report from someone in the ER that "psych had cleared the patient," and they gave the same report to me. No one had taken the time—or *had* the time—to read the actual note to see that further monitoring was recommended, that the patient was still considered suicidal.

Seeing the resident walk by, though, shot an idea into my head. I called Mount Sinai back and asked for the page operator. "This is Dr. Ofri," I said, corralling some authoritative heft into my voice. "Please page the admitting medical resident for me." The operator didn't say a word or even ask if I was a Mount Sinai doctor; she simply patched through what must have been her 1,357th page of the day.

Thirty seconds later a young voice was on the line. I quickly explained that I was a medical attending at Bellevue and that we'd transferred a patient to Mount Sinai this evening. I just needed to confirm that he'd arrived. The resident paused and I could hear clicking on a keyboard. I imagined her scrolling down lists of patients, her mind running down her own scut list, annoyed at this extra task some outside doc had thrust upon her. My foot tapped a jerky syncopation on the floor, and my fingers twisted around themselves in the phone cord. I tried not to think of subway tracks or drugstore shelves.

The resident came back on the line. "How do you spell his name again?"

"Z-H-O-N-G," I said, grabbing clumps of hair in my fist. "First name H-A-O."

"Hmmm, not in the medical department." She paused again. "Computer's really slow tonight," she said, with an edging tone of pleading, clearly hoping I'd thank her for trying and then hang up.

Mr. Zhong's funeral spooled through my head, his grieving family split-screen with a prosecuting attorney in a courtroom. I'd really done it now—let a suicidal patient leave the hospital. How could I be so . . . so . . . stupid? Idiotic? Negligent? Pathetic? Disgraceful? My brain was a veritable thesaurus of culpability.

"Umm, that might be him." The resident interrupted my thoughts. "Did you say Z-H-*O*-N-G or Z-H-*A*-N-G?"

"*O*-N-G," I barked hoarsely into the phone. "Z-H-*O*-N-G." The stiff, cracked vinyl of the chair chafed my thighs. The doctors' station was filled with castoffs from the nurses' station; this one was probably from two renovations ago.

"Wait, here he is," the resident said, a minor note of victory in her otherwise tired voice. "Zhong, Hao. Still in the ER, awaiting a bed on psych."

"But he's there, right?" I said, needing to hear it again before I could register the thought.

"Yeah, he's in the computer system. I can see that he's been admitted to psych already. He's here."

I slumped back in my seat, and the wobbly back of the chair sagged perilously. But I didn't care. The tide of relief insulated me from the usual vertigo that accompanied a recline in the loose-jointed chairs.

We'd avoided the abyss—Mr. Zhong and I—but just narrowly. I whispered an apology aloud. I had endangered his life. It was inexcusable. But the truth was, something like this was inevitable.

The abiding principle on the wards was that since attendings didn't have the time-consuming scut that residents and interns had (drawing blood, placing IVs, chasing down consults, running to radiology), one attending could supervise two teams.

With forty-odd patients and dozens of data points for each patient, there was no possible way I could personally verify every single lab, X-ray, consultation report, physical-exam finding, or progress note for each patient. I relied on verbal reports from my residents for a large percentage of the data. I tried to prioritize and then check on what I thought was the most critical, but the truth was that *anything* could turn out to be critical. When the resident said, "Labs were fine," there could be an unexpectedly low bicarb level within the thirty individual lab values that his statement encompassed. The possibilities for harm seemed endless.

And then there was the time needed to actually evaluate the patients, to talk to them, examine them, read the charts, write my notes. Ten minutes in each patient's room, and then another ten minutes reviewing the chart seemed like a bare minimum. But altogether, that was more than twelve hours right there. And that didn't include rounds, teaching, conferences, let alone grabbing a sandwich or going to the bathroom. Residency regulations limited the number of patients that residents could be in charge of. No such regulations applied to attendings.

Having something slip under the radar was my fear from day one as an attending, and now it had happened. I'm sure many other things slipped under the radar too, but luckily most were benign. Mr. Zhong's episode was a biggie, though it would fall into the near-miss category, since—thankfully—nothing harmful actually transpired. But still, the error was the same, irrespective of the outcome.

A few days later, I related the incident to my colleagues at our weekly meeting, and there were commiserative murmurs all around. The saving grace was that, by and large, all our residents were extremely conscientious—a good thing, since our reliance on them was absolute. Woe to the attending who was assigned to the less compulsive resident.

But I was practicing substandard medicine, and I knew it. The fact that only one major thing had flown under the radar so far was of little comfort. I felt like one of those plate-spinning Chinese acrobats: one plate after another was tossed onto my poles, and I had to keep them all balanced and spinning. If the acrobat dropped one, it was just shattered china to sweep up. If I dropped one, someone could die.

For the rest of the month, I walked around the wards with a film of nervous tension on my skin. What would drop next? I felt as overwhelmed as I had as an intern. Except that as an intern, I always had my resident to turn to. As an attending, there was no one else to pick up my slack. The buck was supposed to stop with me.

A little less than a year after Mr. Zhong slipped from my grasp, things began to change. It became clear that the ratio of one attending to two resident teams was unsustainable and patently unsafe. There needed to be one attending for each resident team. The sticking point was, of course, money. Hiring twice as many attendings was no small budgetary endeavor.

The hospital responded by shifting more doctors from the clinics to the inpatient wards. This helped staff the inpatient side but left the outpatient clinic struggling. Patients had to wait months for appointments, and every one of our sessions in clinic was crammed with overbooked patients. My fear of something flying under the radar simply shifted from my ward months to my clinic months. My amygdala puttered along, unperturbed, steadily feeding my underlying anxieties and fears.

—⁓—

Fears can range from the abject panic of thinking you might have killed your patient through your actions to the low-level worming anxiety that you might be missing something in the everyday care of patients. Some time ago I reviewed a book written by a patient who had a debilitating disease that no doctor could diagnose.[13] The book was part of a series entitled How Patients Think, a complement to (or retaliation for, depending on your perspective) Jerome Groopman's book *How Doctors Think*.

The author wrote of her years of mysterious symptoms that did not fit easily into a simple diagnostic category. Her ailments were labeled psychosomatic (and the author was labeled a "difficult patient"); it took two decades before a correct diagnosis was made. The author turned out to have a rare illness—myasthenia gravis—and this was compounded by the fact that her symptoms were exceedingly atypical for myasthenia. It was a needle in the haystack, and the needle didn't look very much like a needle. This near-impossibility of diagnosis notwithstanding, the patient suffered greatly in the process due to both misdiagnosis and overall poor treatment. Her fury at the medical establishment was palpable.

I read the book attempting to keep the steady, dispassionate eye of a literary reviewer. But it was hard to hold back the bubbling fear of the clinician, of the primary care doctor who sees hundreds of patients with vague, multifaceted, seemingly unrelated symptoms. As I progressed through the pages, I realized that if this patient had come to my office, I surely would have missed the diagnosis too. I would be another in the line of clinicians she writes off—justifiably or not—for blundering her care.

This type of patient is the daily bread of the general practitioners—internists, family doctors, nurse clinicians, physician assistants. In contrast to specialists who have their diseases cut out for them—cardiologists get patients with heart problems, pulmonologists get patients with lung problems—the general practitioner has the far more challenging task of sifting out serious illness from the vast sea of aches and pains that afflict the human race. And this is what we fear, that one of these hundreds of patients will indeed harbor some grave illness and that we will miss it.

Not long ago I wrote an article about one such patient.[14] I described Beverly Wilton as the classic worried-well type of patient—a healthy, fifty-year-old educated white woman with a long litany of nonspecific, unrelated complaints. She was thin and anxious, with tight worry lines carved into her face. When she unfolded a sheet of paper on that Thursday morning with a brisk snap, my heart sank as I saw thirty lines of hand-printed concerns. Ms. Wilton, like Mrs. Alvarez, is the type of patient who can overwhelm a doctor, quickly siphoning off reserves of time, clinical reasoning, and empathy.

Ms. Wilton told me that she had recently started smoking again after her elderly mother became ill, and she was up to a pack a day now. She had headaches, eye pain, abdominal pain, pounding in her ears, shortness of breath, and dizziness. She experienced dryness when she swallowed, needling sensations in her chest, tightness in her gut. She couldn't fall asleep at night. And she really, really wanted a cigarette, she told me, nervously eyeing the door.

This is the patient who makes me feel as though I'm drowning. I avoid asking the comprehensive review-of-systems questions because I know I'll get a yes to everything.

When I teach residents and medical students, I always ask them to place a patient's symptoms within a physiologic paradigm. Most diseases have specific symptoms, related to the particular pathology at hand. There are certainly illnesses with global symptoms—many endocrine and rheumatologic diseases, for example—but even these diseases usually have recognizable patterns.

For most patients, if they *truly* have significant organic pathology of the renal, neurologic, gastrointestinal, pulmonary, and cardiac systems simultaneously, they are devastatingly ill and not hard to miss.

But the overwhelming majority of patients who come to an outpatient medical clinic with multitudes of symptoms are like the patient who sat before me on this day—healthy-appearing, with a good exercise capacity, stable weight, and a perfectly normal physical exam. Ms. Wilton even had a normal EKG and cardiac stress test done within the past year. It would be exceedingly unlikely for a serious illness affecting multiple organs to be present in this sort of patient.

The metaphor of drowning is not only apt; it's diagnostic. It is a clue that something else may be going on, that the doctor needs to probe for other issues, such as stress, depression, domestic violence, eating disorders. When I administered a questionnaire for anxiety and depression, Ms. Wilton selected the highest value for every question.

I told her that her symptoms were most likely from anxiety and Ms. Wilton seemed relieved. "My mother is impossible," she said. "I try to be there for her while she's sick, but she is just as crabby as always. In fact, that's the first time I ever got chest pains—when I visited her after her surgery last month. The same thing happened with I visited her at rehab last week."

She brought her fingers to her temples and squeezed a cage around her face. "Every time I take off from work to get her to the doctor, I get flak from my boss. And my son, he's twenty-eight, but he still can't support himself. No wonder I'm smoking like a chimney."

I could envision the vise-like tension pressing in from every facet of her life. I explained how stress could cause physical symptoms, and though we couldn't change the facts of her life, we could try to ease the pain by treating some of the symptoms of stress. Ms. Wilton welcomed this approach, and I felt a sense of satisfaction that I might actually be helping my patient where she really needed it.

Fourteen hours later, in the dead of night, my pager went off: extension 3015. The emergency room. Never a good sign. I called in and got the news from an intern. Ms. Wilton had been admitted to the hospital with a pulmonary embolus—a blood clot in the lung.

A pulmonary embolus, a leading cause of sudden death—it was hard to get much worse than that. I sank down onto a chair, clenching my eyes against the stinging ray of guilt. My worst fear had come true: a patient with vague and seemingly unrelated symptoms turned out to have a life-threatening illness. As the intern spoke, my mind raked back over my encounter with Ms. Wilton, all the symptoms she had listed for me.

There they were—chest pain and shortness of breath—buried in her sea of anxiety, job worries, family concerns. A potentially fatal condition was right smack in front of me as I prescribed her sleeping pills and a visit to a psychiatrist.

"Oh, and it was bilateral," the intern added. I sank my chin against my chest, too traumatized to reply. The presence of blood clots in both lungs meant that she'd be sentenced to a lifetime of blood thinners to prevent future clots. No one wants to take a chance with bilateral pulmonary emboli.

Ms. Wilton had fit the stereotype of the worried well so perfectly. Her expansive and multifaceted list of complaints was classic for a person suffering from emotional stress. Occam's razor—the law of diagnostic parsimony—tells us that the simpler explanation, the single condition, usually underlies the patient's symptoms.

However, there is the counterargument, Hickam's dictum, which states, in essence, that patients can have as many diseases as they damn well please. Ms. Wilton did indeed suffer from emotional stress and had many symptoms resulting from that. But at the moment she sat in my office, she also had a handful of blood clots growing inside her.

It's Hickam's dictum that terrifies doctors: even when you think you've made the most reasonable diagnosis, there could be something else lurking, something horrific. If you make that sort of error while picking stocks for investment, or filling out a 1040, you might lose a little money. Or a lot of money. Or a lot of clients. But you won't kill someone. This fear is the inner lining of a doctor's daily life.

After reading Jerome Groopman's book *How Doctors Think*[15]— which filled me with plenty more fears of the myriad errors I could be making—I tried to analyze the cognitive errors that led to my misdiagnosis. For Ms. Wilton, her shortness of breath blended into the greater landscape of her many symptoms. This symptom did not stand out in terms of severity or time course. Plus, it seemed to occur only when she visited her mother. This blending of symptoms was mirrored in my mind as well. Not to mention my attribution bias, which my judgment solidified around my stereotype of a healthy-appearing, educated white female with an extensively prepared list of complaints.

How might I have picked up on the pulmonary embolism? The brute-force approach might have dug the needle from the haystack. If I had taken every symptom in isolation and asked—as every medical student is taught to do—about duration, severity, provoking and relieving factors, associated symptoms, I might have found the shortness of breath to be the key symptom.

The truth is, any one of her symptoms might have masked a life-threatening illness and could have justified a full medical investigation: Headaches could have been a cerebral aneurysm. Abdominal pain could have been a bleeding ulcer. Needling sensations in the chest could have been angina.

Dissecting each symptom in isolation with textbook-perfect detail would have taken easily an hour or more. This technique works heroically well in books, movies, and clinical legends, but in real life there is a waiting room full of patients, all of whom could rightfully complain that their doctor was arrogantly ignoring them and taking their time for granted. And of course, in this era of accountability and quality measures, I would have been dinged for being inefficient and not meeting "productivity goals."

In the real world, I had twenty minutes allotted to evaluate, treat, and document Ms. Wilton's myriad symptoms. I performed my history and my physical exam, and then I relied on my instinct that it was extremely unlikely that Ms. Wilton had a cerebral aneurysm *and* a bleeding ulcer *and* angina *and* a pulmonary embolus. She couldn't have all that and look as well as she did.

I relied on my experience, my clinical judgment, as well as my stereotyping, and chalked it all up to stress. And I was wrong. My fears about harming patients, fears that had been tamped down somewhat with my years of experience—and perhaps simple good fortune—reignited with a vengeance.

When I wrote the article about her case, my original intent had been to examine the role of stereotyping in medicine, pointing out that I'd even managed to stereotype myself—white, educated, female, neurotic. What I wasn't prepared for were the scathing reader comments that were posted online. *How could you be so incompetent? Doctors never listen to their patients! Those arrogant doctors never take the time to hear the full story! Those money-grubbing doctors are just milking the system!*

It was dispiriting, to say the least, especially because I thought I *had* taken the time to listen to Ms. Wilton's story, to tease out the context of her life that might have affected her illness. I realized that I would probably make the same mistake again, that I would likely miss a pulmonary embolism, just like I would have no doubt missed the myasthenia gravis of the patient who wrote the book I had reviewed. Just as I might miss a serious problem in Mrs. Alvarez next time she appears with her host of "worst-ever" symptoms.

Despite my years of experience, despite my training, despite my diligence, there is no doubt that I will make more mistakes in the future, that I might harm a patient, that I could easily get battered in a lawsuit. Maybe—and here, perhaps, is the deepest existential fear—I simply am not good enough to be a doctor. Maybe I need to take down my shingle and let my patients be cared for by more competent hands.

But as I look around at my colleagues, I think that I fall within the acceptable range of capability, that I'm probably not much worse or much better than they. When I started speaking to them, I realized that they all carried around this same fear—fear of harming patients, fear of not being good enough. One of my colleagues summed it up only half jokingly, saying, "Every day is an opportunity to lose our license."

She recalled a time when her mind wandered for a brief moment while an intern plodded through a case presentation. It was one of twenty such cases she'd been listening to all afternoon, each one presented in a droning monotone. The day was growing late, and she was thinking that she could use another cup of coffee. Nevertheless, she jogged herself back into focus, just as the intern was saying something about a patient's foot looking a little dusky so he was going to give the patient a podiatry appointment for two weeks hence. That was when her own inner caffeine jolted her upright.

A *dusky foot* is one of those heart-stopping terms in medicine, because it can mean a limb is losing blood flow. For these patients— who usually have diabetes and severe vascular disease—that limb might need emergency surgical treatment to restore blood flow. Or, if the lack of blood has already done too much damage, then the limb might have to be amputated promptly to avoid deadly gangrene. This kind of patient needs to see a vascular surgeon immediately to gauge the severity of the situation, not a podiatrist in two weeks. A dusky foot could certainly turn out to be nothing more than discolored skin, but it's not something you take a chance with.

The intern hadn't understood the gravity of the situation and so was doing what he thought was reasonable. But for the attending, her momentary lapse of attention was terrifying. A few seconds longer and that patient's dusky foot would have disappeared into the haze of vaccinations, mammograms, and other nonurgent matters. If the blood supply had indeed been compromised, the patient could have lost his leg, or his life.

I visited Ms. Wilton in the hospital the following day. Her breathing was better, thanks to the timely treatment she'd received in the ER. We talked about the gravity of a pulmonary embolus and the need for her to take blood thinners for the rest of her life to prevent recurrence. However, too high a dose of blood thinners could cause bleeding; too low could allow another blood clot. From this day onward, Ms. Wilton would have to live in the precariously narrow canyon between clotting and bleeding, teetering forever between the risks of pulmonary embolism and the risks of bleeding ulcers or strokes, all of which could be deadly. I had to own up.

"I need to offer you an apology," I said, my voice slackening. "I missed this diagnosis. You told me about your shortness of breath and your chest pain. But given all your other symptoms, I didn't think of a blood clot in your lungs." The mere articulation of these words was agonizing. The concise summary seemed only to concretize the fact that my actions could very well have killed Ms. Wilton.

Sudden death is frequently, in fact, one of the first symptoms of pulmonary embolism. "I . . . I'm sorry."

Ms. Wilton waved her hand dismissively. "The truth is," she said, "I didn't think anything of the chest pains either. I'd had this appointment scheduled with you for months—way before the chest pains started—so I guess it was just random chance that this blood clot happened now."

I appreciated her forgiveness. The random timing of the embolus offered some comfort, as did the knowledge that pulmonary embolism is known to be a notoriously difficult disease to diagnose. But I realized that not only did I need to keep tuning my skills as a doctor, I also had to figure out a way to live with the uncertainty of medicine and its attendant anxiety. As sure as the sun will rise, as sure as the next ambulance will roll into the ER, as sure as the next patient will walk into a doctor's office with a list of vague symptoms, mistakes will happen. From autopsies, it is estimated that 10 to 15 percent of diagnoses are incorrect.[16] There is an entire academic field devoted to studying diagnostic reasoning and how to decrease errors in our thought processes.[17] But this research doesn't address the issue of how individual doctors incorporate the ongoing prickly thrum of discomfort inherent in this imperfect science of medicine.

After Ms. Wilton, I reconsidered my approach to the patient with a sea of complaints. When a patient presents with so many complaints that it's not possible to cover them all in depth, I now openly acknowledge to her that impossibility. But then I say, "Today, we are going to review three of your concerns: you pick two, and I'll pick one." This allows the patient to select the two most concerning issues, and allows me to home in on the one I think might conceal a serious illness. And then after I reach a conclusion, I remind myself to go back and ask, "Could it be anything else? Is there something I might have missed?"

This approach may improve my diagnostic accuracy, but it doesn't curtail the fear that percolates in the background of every encounter, keeping me on edge, never allowing me to feel perfectly at ease with being a doctor. In Ernest Becker's view, humans use denial to erase the palpability of death in such a way that we don't even realize that we are reacting to this existential fear. But in medicine, that layer of denial is curled back just enough to let us be consciously aware of it.

For that, I can only take a deep breath and acknowledge to myself that this is not an aberration, but an integral part of clinical medicine. Being a doctor means living with that fear, incorporating it into one's daily life. It is like stepping onto a moving carousel and feeling your stomach drop, yet needing to continue forward despite the queasiness.

There's no easy answer about how to proceed onward in daily medical life with that ongoing churn of anxiety and fear, and certainly no research to guide us. Each doctor has to come to terms with it and negotiate an individual emotional armistice. We need to keep it nestled in a recess contained enough to permit us to function. But if we wall it off too hermetically, we will lose a fundamental layer in the polyphonic texture of being a doctor. This fear and anxiety, in a modest amount, maintains the reverential and vigilant stratum required in caring for other human beings. We physicians need to tuck it away but also keep it alive.

When I was a patient—giving birth to one of my children—I had a doctor known for his warm bedside manner. Everybody loved him. He was covering for my regular OB that day, but I was comfortable with that since I'd met him before. He was cheerful and warm and I felt that I was in good hands. Things were moving along swimmingly until suddenly they weren't. The fetal heart monitor showed concerning late decelerations, and the pH wasn't where it should have been.

I remember distinctly how his manner changed. The pleasant cheer melted away and a tense focus replaced it. Small talk vanished. It didn't feel like his prior congeniality had been fake, but now I had a sense of his concern and fear coming through as he checked a second pH, and then a third when the first two conflicted. I was anxious, to be sure, terrified, but in an odd way, something about sensing the doctor's fear reassured me. He was taking nothing for granted. When he called in a second doctor for assistance, I could feel his growing anxiety.

As a patient, I *wanted* my doctor to be scared, just a bit, just enough to ground him in the profound weight of what he was doing. I obviously didn't want him to be overwhelmed, but at that moment, I had no way of controlling the outcome. I was ceding the fate of my child to this doctor and I wanted him to feel the fearful awe—in the truest sense of the word—for the life-and-death side of medicine.

Fear, like all emotions, is neither good nor bad; it is simply one of the normal states of being. Overwhelming fear can be incapacitating, as I learned during my first code. But appropriate fear, as I witnessed in my obstetrician, can be crucial for good medical care, especially during critical situations. All eventually worked out well for me and my baby, but I gained an appreciation for how fear in the right dose might serve the doctor—and the patient—well. Being aware of our fear and figuring out how to titrate it appropriately is a vital skill for a doctor. Our patients' lives may depend on it.

Julia, part three

Julia spent several weeks in the Bellevue ICU after our encounter that fall morning. She was placed on high-dose diuretics to ease the pressure on her heart, which unfortunately eased her blood pressure down to zilch. Powerful intravenous pressors (adrenaline-like medications) were required to keep her blood pressure at survival levels.

For the first week, she hovered on the edge of death. Whenever we attempted to lower the dosage of the pressors, her blood pressure plummeted to 60/40, not enough to keep her brain and kidneys functioning. So the pressors remained at high doses. But pressors are no free lunch—they can overly constrict the blood supply to the heart muscle and kidneys, they can cause arrhythmias, push the heart into overdrive, not to mention that the patient is tethered to an IV in an intensive care unit every waking (and sleeping) minute.

Normally, when a patient hits the point that her heart can function only while on pressors in an ICU, it's time for the heart transplant. But of course, that wasn't on our list of options. I could hardly bring myself to think of what would happen next. Would Julia just stay in the ICU until the pressors caused some horrific side effect, forcing us to turn them off? Then would we just wait until her heart ran itself down? I blocked all of this out of my mind, focusing only on the minute-to-minute of her vital signs.

It was touch-and-go, but haltingly, amazingly, Julia's heart clawed its way up from the depths. It never returned to its previous equilibrium, the one that offered me such easy denial, but it settled at a survivable station. Over the ensuing weeks, the diuretics and pressors were gingerly weaned. Every few days there would be a setback and we'd have to start again, but with the painstaking efforts of Julia and the medical staff, she made it out of the ICU. She spent another week on the regular medical ward, and then two weeks in cardiac rehab, but finally she went home. Julia was severely weakened, but she was alive. A stay of execution had been granted, and we were both acutely cognizant of that.

Julia convalesced at home within the circle of her family and close friends as well as in the framework of her otherwise healthy body. She never returned to her earlier condition, but she did regain some of her health. She was slower now, more tentative, but a bloom eventually returned to her face. The winter was tenuous, but she held on, still taking her medications with religious fervor, still making the long trip from Brooklyn to Manhattan for every appointment. She had recently separated from her husband but seemed to be on solid emotional ground with this. Her sister was pitching in with the kids, and the two of them were keeping the family together.

I had just finalized the manuscript of *Medicine in Translation* when a spring snowstorm hit New York City that March. A foot of snow blanketed the city, and Manhattan resembled a winter scene from *Little House on the Prairie*. While my children reveled in the snow day off from school, I trudged the slushy blocks to Bellevue, wishing I owned cross-country skis.

It was startling how many of my patients arrived for their appointments despite the arctic weather. And there was Julia, cheeks glowing crimson from the cold. How she made it through the snow I'll never know, but she did. Her resilient body was fighting back, as was her spirit. She talked about *esperanza*—hope—and I could feel myself being pulled into that optimistic orbit, despite my intellectual knowledge that this was foolhardy. We hugged tightly that day, and it felt so good to allow her buoyancy to peel me away from the facts on the ground.

Maybe everything *would* be okay. I'd just witnessed Julia beat death at its own game, after all. Maybe she was that rare biological exception to the rule, the exception that confounded the rules. Why not? When she left my office, I was convinced that somehow it would all work out. I couldn't say how, but I was sure that it would.

I reopened my manuscript and furiously typed a new ending to *Medicine in Translation*. Snowstorm, redemption, hope—that was the right ending note for the book.

CHAPTER 4

A Daily Dose of Death

One of the most frequent questions I'm asked by people outside the medical field is how doctors handle all the sickness, suffering, and death. "Isn't it so depressing?" they usually say. All fields have occupational hazards, and for medicine, sadness is certainly one of them. Like fear, sadness is neither good nor bad; it is simply a component of the human condition. What matters is how the sadness is navigated, something that is influenced by both the individual personality of the doctor and the surrounding environment. There are some doctors who appear particularly skilled at not letting the suffering and pain get to them. They seem impervious.

There were times in my training when I envied those doctors, when I wished my armor were stronger. But I also grew to learn that this armor could be destructive, as it does not actually prevent grief from entering; it only channels it into an awkward holding area. Somehow, some way, all of this eventually burrows within us, powerfully affecting how we take care of our future patients. How can it not? Grief is one of the most commanding of human emotions, and it does not tread lightly.

Eva, a pediatrician I interviewed extensively for this book, shared experiences that potently illustrate the depth to which sorrow can affect medical care.

It was just the beginning of her night on call when Eva was paged to the delivery room: labor had started. Midway through her pediatrics internship, Eva had already attended dozens of deliveries. But this one came with an explicit warning: "The parents do not want to see the baby."

Dashing up to the Labor and Delivery suite to meet her resident, Eric, Eva reviewed in her head what she recalled about Potter syndrome. A severe lack of amniotic fluid due to damaged fetal kidneys was the primary problem. But the main fallout was that the lungs couldn't develop properly without sufficient amniotic fluid. Nearly every baby born with Potter syndrome was doomed to death by asphyxiation within minutes of birth.

She met up with Eric—two years her senior—outside the labor room. Neither said a word, but Eva caught his expression—a mixture of exhaustion, disdain, and harriedness. It was clear he'd rather be anywhere but there. Wordlessly, they scrubbed, gowned, and entered. There were already six people crowded into the cramped delivery room, but it was eerily quiet. The windows were blackened by the night, and the desolation of the Vermont winter seemed to have infused the room.

When Eva had interviewed for residency fifteen months earlier, it was the beginning of October, and the foliage was a ravishing array of gold and vermilion. To someone who'd spent the past decade in the spare dustscapes of New Mexico, the lush New England autumn was intoxicating. But all was barren now. The bleakness of winter and the brutal months of training had taken their toll on the entire class of interns.

Eva took a deep breath and pulled herself together for the task at hand. Her irrational first thought was *Where are the parents?* The mother on the delivery table and the father standing next to her didn't look old enough to buy a beer in a Burlington bar, maybe not even old enough to vote. The boy cradled the girl's head in his arms, shielding her line of vision. Apparently they'd been told that the baby would look strange, and it was clear from their body language that they didn't want to see any of what was going on. Eva didn't know any details about them, but she guessed they were unmarried, working-class teenagers, that this was an unexpected pregnancy, that they were completely unprepared to be thrust into the stormy seas of high-risk neonatology. She had a flash of sympathy for their decision not to see the baby. It was probably all too overwhelming.

The obstetrics team paid dogged attention to the business end of the delivery. So did the pediatrics team. The parents were determinedly focusing anywhere but down. Nobody uttered a word.

The delivery proceeded normally. No complications. When the baby emerged, it was greeted with muteness. No "Congratulations!" No "It's a girl!" Just leaden silence as the baby was passed off from obstetrics to pediatrics. Eva quickly wrapped the baby in a blanket. It felt floppy, like a rag doll. But Eva did not have time to meditate on this.

She and Eric hurried out of the room as they had been instructed to do. Once in the hall, they suddenly stopped short, wondering where they were supposed to go with this baby who was dying but wouldn't be—couldn't be—resuscitated. Eva grasped the bundle to her chest as Eric madly scanned the delivery board. Every room was occupied. They scurried over to the postpartum ward, but every room there was taken.

They stood stranded in the hallway, dying baby in tow, as it became clear there was nowhere to go. Eric's fingers were jittering and Eva knew he was dying for a cigarette. He finally grabbed the door to a supply closet at the end of the hall and hustled Eva and the baby inside. At least it was empty.

They crowded into the tiny closet that was overflowing with shelves of surgical instruments, bags of saline, IVs, blood tubes, and urine cups. An unused incubator was crammed into the tiny space, along with a squat metal supply cart. Eva and Eric squeezed themselves into the few inches between the incubator and the cart and glanced around for a place to examine the baby. The supply cart was the only flat space available. Eric moved aside the boxes of gloves on the cart, and Eva gingerly laid the baby down.

Slowly she undid the blanket. The baby's face was gray-blue, stubby and crumpled from the lack of space in a uterus deprived of amniotic fluid. The ears were low-set, a classic sign of fetal abnormalities. "Blueberry-muffin" skin hinted at bleeding beneath the skin.

The baby's mouth puckered with a futile gasp at air. Then it gave a second, wispier attempt. Then it stilled. Eva looked nervously at Eric. He was silent a full minute, then said to Eva, "You need to record the time of death."

Eva had a moment of panic. Did this count as the moment of death, when the baby stopped breathing? Eric gave a nod to her stethoscope, and she tugged it out and hurriedly placed the tiny bell on the baby's rubbery chest. Were those faint *bup*s actual heart sounds, or was she imagining them? Or was she just hearing her own heart pounding in her ears?

"I remember feeling incredibly stupid for not knowing whether the baby was dead or not," Eva recalled. "I mean, isn't that the most basic thing a doctor should be able to tell you, whether the patient is alive or dead?"

Eric rolled his eyes and pointed at the umbilical cord that was still pulsating, indicating a pumping heart. In Potter syndrome, the lungs are abnormal, but the heart is not. The heart would keep beating until the lack of oxygen finally starved the cardiac muscle to death. "Record when the umbilical cord stops pulsing," Eric instructed, and then he disappeared out the door.

Drilled into the head of every pediatrics resident are the protocols of newborn resuscitation. The first, most crucial step is to keep the baby warm. It went against Eva's every impulse to leave a newborn lying on a cold metal surface.

"I felt guilty not doing anything to keep this baby alive," Eva said, "but if I wrapped the blanket tight to keep in the warmth, the heart might keep beating longer. And I wouldn't be able to see when the umbilical cord stopped pulsating. And I would be stuck in this closet with a dysmorphic, dying baby for longer."

As she stood there, staring at this baby lying limp on the frigid metal cart, Eva wondered what she would have done had she been in the mother's situation. How painful it would be to have this baby growing inside you, knowing that it was going to die as soon as it came out.

Eva was suddenly consumed with a wave of immense sadness for this tiny baby, this little girl. To never have been held by her parents, to never have been held by anyone. It was almost beyond comprehension.

Knowing she'd surely be reprimanded for not observing the precise moment of umbilical-pulse cessation, Eva gathered the blankets around the baby's rigid body. She scooped the fragile girl into her arms and leaned back against a shelf of saline bottles. In the cramped space Eva rocked back and forth. "I love you, baby," she whispered as the heart began its slow, cratering descent. "I love you."

Dying is not slow when you are watching it in real time. Eva kept rocking as the pulse ratcheted reluctantly down, surprisingly stalwart despite the lack of oxygen. Five minutes. Ten minutes. Fifteen minutes. Finally all was still.

Stiff from standing in one position for so long, Eva pushed the closet door open and emerged into the overly bright hallway. She shuffled numbly toward the nursing station, still gripping the bundled baby. When she saw Eric by the chart rack, he reminded her to fill out the paperwork. "Oh, and don't forget to call the morgue," he added as he dashed down the hall, checking the number on his beeper. It was only the beginning of their night on call, and the cases were backing up.

Eva had no idea how to call the morgue or where to find it; she hadn't had to deal with the morgue thus far in her pediatrics residency. Finally, she turned to a nurse, who knew the phone number off the top of her head. The nurses had seen it all before, but for Eva it was a first. Babies could die.

Eva doesn't quite remember how she made it through the rest of the night, but she did. She had to. It was just her and Eric, responsible for every zero- to eighteen-year-old in the entire hospital during the night. She plowed through the next day as well, rounding on the neonatal ICU preemies and the gravely ill children who made up the inpatient pediatric ward of the teaching hospital—the only teaching hospital in the entire state. "I guess I just stuffed the whole thing way down in my consciousness."

All of residency seemed to be an exercise in stuffing traumatic experiences way down in the consciousness. There just wasn't time, space, or emotional energy to delve into how these experiences were affecting the residents. And, certainly, the institutional environment did not exude an openness to hearing about such issues.

By the end of residency, Eva was focused only on survival, on holding everything together. Two weeks before her final day of residency, a four-year-old boy was rushed to the hospital by ambulance after drowning in a lake. The pediatrics team flew into action to resuscitate him.

A code in pediatrics has a completely different feeling from a code in adult medicine. The codes that we internists participate in tend to be of elderly, critically ill patients with a host of medical misfortunes that nearly guarantee the code's failure. The majority of times we start a code, we know it's futile.

In pediatrics, though, it is a child before you, with seventy, eighty, or ninety years of life waiting ahead, so the stakes are higher. Also, most codes in pediatrics are not of critically ill patients; they are of healthy patients—like this little boy—who have stopped breathing because of choking or drowning. Their hearts, lungs, kidneys, and brains are in pristine condition, and if the breathing can be restored promptly, these children will live perfectly healthy, long lives.

Unless, of course, the choking or drowning has lasted a bit too long. Within seconds of a brain's losing oxygen, there is damage. Within a minute or two, brain cells are dying off. After five minutes, there is permanent damage. After ten minutes, there is virtually no hope of survival. Children's bodies, however, tend to be more resilient than adults', and pediatricians cling to this thread of hope during a code.

Eva's team did successfully resuscitate this boy, or, rather, they successfully resuscitated his body. Breathing and circulation were restored, but it was too late for the brain.

For the final two weeks of her residency, Eva dutifully tended the body of this comatose child in the ICU. The boy's silky blond hair, blue eyes, and angelic face were perfectly maintained. It was a tragic case with palpable anguish everywhere, but Eva did not feel even a twinge of emotion.

The family had been visiting from Texas, staying at a fancy lakeside resort for a wedding. The mother and son were standing together on the pier. When the mother zipped inside to use the bathroom, the son tumbled into the icy, unforgiving waters of Lake Champlain. But Eva did not shed a single tear, even when she heard the spine-chilling wail—"I'm . . . a . . . terrible . . . mother"—followed by choking sobs that echoed throughout the ICU. Eva's armor had solidified.

Every day the family would bring in more photos of the boy and post them in his room. The family was well-to-do, and the pictures showed a sparkling boy frolicking on an expansive lawn, trotting on his pony, relaxing on the family boat. "Goddamn it," Eva would mutter to herself every time she entered the room and saw another idyllic picture pasted up, "don't make him into a real boy."

"I wanted to keep him as just a set of electrolytes to keep in line," Eva said. "Just vent settings I had to adjust." Anything to avoid feeling. The mother, however, was constantly trying to engage Eva in conversation about her boy, about the real person that he was. "He loved to speak French," she would say. "Soccer was his favorite sport." Eva avoided the room as much as possible.

"I felt absolutely nothing for that boy and his family during the entire two weeks I cared for him," she recalled. "I was almost finished with residency, almost out of this mess where I was always dealing with dead or near-dead children. I was determined that this was not going to bring me down."

But this wasn't easy. Next door to the drowned boy was a three-month-old preemie. Her three months of life had been extremely rocky, and the baby had suffered endless complications. When the baby coded, the team worked furiously to save her, but they were stymied by a lack of IV access. (Veins in babies are hair-thin; veins in preemies, microscopic.) The code wore on, and the team became frantic. As a last-ditch effort, Eva stabbed a syringe of epinephrine directly into the baby's heart. Miraculously, the pulse returned. Breathing was restored. But when Eva looked up at the clock, fifteen minutes had elapsed. Once again, a body had been resuscitated without any of the person who inhabited the body.

When Eva reviewed the code with the mother, she explained about the intracardiac injection and how it had restored the vital signs but not the neurological function. The mother's anguished response was "Why did you do that?"

At first Eva was stunned by the reaction—she had saved the baby, after all. But then she realized that she had just sentenced the mother to a lifetime of hell, of caring for a vegetative body that would never recover. Eva wished she could take it back, undo the injection that would prolong the family's nightmare. She wished she'd allowed the baby to die. But here they were, inhabiting the grotesque reality of the NICU, with no escape.

Eva knew she needed to break away from the world of critically ill children, so she decided to pursue child psychiatry after her pediatrics residency ended. Child psychiatry, however, entailed enrolling in an adult-psychiatry residency first.

"I went from treating innocent babes to treating ax murderers," was how Eva put it. One of her patients—recently released from Rikers Island jail—stalked up and down the halls muttering, "I didn't rape that woman. I didn't rape her." It turned out that he hadn't, in fact, been incarcerated for rape but rather for planting an ax in his social worker's head when she hadn't gotten his disability check to him fast enough.

Eva's reserve of empathy was entirely empty by now. Once she was paged at 3:00 a.m. to check that an alcoholic who had fallen out of his hospital bed had not sustained any head trauma. She went through the motions of examining the patient and ordering a head CT, but she realized that she didn't care one way or another. "At that moment, I really didn't give a fuck whether he was bleeding in his head," she said. That was when she realized that she couldn't go on like this anymore. She quit the psychiatry residency midway through her first year and "went into hibernation" for the next three months.

One day during that hibernation, Eva attended a movie matinee, a decadence she hadn't indulged in since childhood. She went by herself, just to veg out at a lighthearted Hollywood flick. In the middle of the movie, there was a scene of a child languidly drifting down into deep water. Little bubbles percolated from her mouth as the oxygen steadily escaped. The child's hair billowed lazily from her face, illuminated by the water-refracted sun. Of course, the character wasn't really drowning; the movie was a comedy, after all. But as Eva watched, the girl sank lower and lower, a relentless descent in agonizing slow motion. It was almost as though Eva could see the girl's EKG gradually flattening out as the lack of oxygen extinguished the heart.

A shudder of emotion hit Eva with bodily force. In seconds, she was sobbing uncontrollably, her body trembling in the plush velvet seat. In a rush it all came back—the blond, blue-eyed boy who had drowned, the mother's piercing wails of anguish after the code, the inert body kept alive on a ventilator. She searched madly in her pockets for tissues, but she had none.

She bunched her sleeves against her eyes, trying to stanch the flow. The movie had already moved on to some silly scene, but Eva was still bawling. What would the other people in the audience think?

It was exactly like posttraumatic stress disorder experienced by war veterans—a single sight or sound could allow a flood of harrowing memories to break through the dam of protection honed so assiduously by the soul.

Eva's residency truly was a traumatic experience in which survival was the mode of operation. And the PTSD that resulted was real. Classic PTSD is marked by nightmares, flashbacks, emotional numbing, and exaggerated startle response. Eva had experienced them all. She described a nightmare she once had that she herself was a preemie, strapped down with lights blinding her eyes, people stabbing at her with IVs, chest tubes, endotracheal tubes, umbilical catheters. (She often wonders whether these preemies themselves experience some form of PTSD from all the trauma they have endured.)

"For years after residency," she says, "the sound of a beeper going off would immediately make my heart jump. Instant fight-or-flight." Even when she was in private practice much later, when the sound of her beeper meant only that she had to return a phone call, not resuscitate a dying child, it would still make her nerves clench.

What struck me in listening to Eva's experiences was the simultaneous presence and absence of grief. The profound sadness of dying babies, mourning parents, vegetative children is impossible to ignore.

Yet the culture of medicine doesn't offer much space to explore this. Certainly, in the breakneck pace of Eva's residency, there was barely a blip of acknowledgment for the wells of sadness that bloomed, day after day. It's no wonder that her emotions finally erupted as she sat in the movie theater.

Grief is an overwhelming emotion for anyone who faces tragedy, so it is surprising how little attention it receives in medicine, where death is a more regular occurrence than in most any other profession. One of the few studies that has looked in depth at the nature and impact of grief on physicians centered on oncologists.[1] Oncology, by its nature, counts death as part and parcel of its daily routine. Despite the enormous therapeutic advances in the field, cancer is still an arena where death's presence is palpable and prominent. The extensive interviews with oncologists confirmed this: grief was pervasive in their lives.

Nearly every single doctor in the study spoke of compartmentalizing the sadness to keep it separate from their daily work and their personal lives. The most striking finding of the study was how poorly that strategy worked. Grief, the authors wrote, "was pervasive, sticking to the physicians' clothes when they went home after work and slipping under the doors between patient rooms."

Grief had a profound effect on these doctors, spilling into their personal lives and depleting their inner reserves of strength. "It's a physical sensation of being ground away," said one physician, who was facing one or two deaths each week. "It takes me a long time to recover from that."

The pervasiveness of death often led to a relentless sense of grief among the oncologists, not just for the patients who had died but for the patients whom they knew would be dying soon. "I go through weeks where it's very difficult to come into work," another doctor said, "because I know that I'm going to see patients who are going to do badly."

Grief ate at these doctors, distracting them from both their families and their patients. Many reported withdrawing from emotional involvement with their patients and that their patients had noticed they weren't fully present.

Most significantly for health care, the presence of this grief directly affected how these doctors cared for their patients. Some doctors reported that after a death that felt to them like a "failure," they would treat the next few patients overaggressively. Conversely, if doctors had witnessed what seemed like unnecessary suffering, they would pull back with the next few patients, leaning away from aggressive treatment, even when it might have been warranted.

This is not to say that grief is bad. On the contrary, it is a primal emotion that is a defining characteristic of humanity. In this study of oncologists, many doctors acknowledged that grief offered perspective on life, and a dose of humility about the limits of medicine. For many, it redoubled their commitment to medicine, enhanced their appreciation of family and good health. The doctors did not at all want to erase the grief about their patients; they were cognizant that their ability to feel sad was critical to maintaining who they were. But there was clearly a need to do something with this emotional omnipresence, to engage it somehow so that it integrated into their lives instead of overpowering their lives.

Sadness and grief will never leave medicine, and, of course, it shouldn't. Illness and death are integral aspects of medicine, and if there were no sadness or grief in response, then we would just be robots dispensing prescriptions. The problem, as Eva's story illustrates, is that the grief is largely unacknowledged. With no time or space to give grief its due, burnout, callousness, PTSD, and skewed treatment decisions are a risk.

The medical field is slowly beginning to address this. At the University of Rochester, a staff support group meets regularly, facilitated jointly by an oncology physician, an expert in palliative care, and a representative from the chaplaincy.[2] The group is open to anyone who works with cancer patients, from secretaries to social workers to nurses to senior physicians. But it is mandatory for the oncology fellows, the oncologists-in-training. Making the group a requirement for the fellows—just as they are required to attend conferences, grand rounds, and clinics—sends a clear message that engaging the emotional side of medicine is a critical pillar of medical training, not optional fluff. It affects not just the doctor you are but also the person you are.

The support group allows participants to discuss issues they have been wrestling with, particularly in regard to patient loss and grief. People share coping strategies, and there is an emphasis on self-care. Attending to personal needs is not considered selfish; rather, it is something that responsible doctors do in order to take the best care of their patients. And, importantly, there is time set aside to acknowledge the patients who have died. Participants can offer up the names of the patients whom they've lost, and a moment of silence is shared by the group.

I wonder how things might have worked out for Eva if she'd had this sort of support during her pediatrics residency. If skilled and compassionate higher-ups had taken the time to explore what it meant for a young intern to watch a doomed newborn die in her arms, she might have been better equipped to help the mother of the young boy who had drowned. If the program had offered its trainees space to acknowledge the intense emotions precipitated by these situations, Eva might not have experienced the explosion of PTSD in the movie theater.

Eva now works in a general pediatrics practice, and the pace of life is much calmer. No preemies coding, no children dying of cancer, no babies on ventilators. The transition from the residency mindset, however, was stark, somewhat akin to being parachuted into another solar system. "When I finished residency I could tell you from memory how many cc/kg/day of fluids to give a twenty-four-weeker," she says. "I could administer intrathecal [in the spinal column] chemotherapy with one hand tied behind my back. But ask me a question about toilet training or how to get a baby to sleep through the night and I was like a deer caught in the headlights."

Eventually she came to know the ins and outs of general pediatrics, how to settle parents' anxiety about teething, diaper rash, and infant formula. There was something soothing about the prosaic rhythm of vaccinations and school physicals. *Sick* meant a sore throat or an ear infection, not a leukemic blast crisis. This was the beauty of general pediatrics—even if you did nothing, just about everything got better.

But the experiences of residency nested within her, informing how she acted as a doctor. Many years later, Eva attended the delivery of an infant with Apert syndrome. Babies with Apert syndrome have serious deformities of the face and skull. Fingers and toes are fused together like mittens. Unlike Potter syndrome, however, there is no immediate threat to life. Babies with Apert syndrome will require many surgeries in early childhood to correct the deformities, but generally there is no imminent danger at birth.

In this instance, the family was prepared. The parents knew what the baby would look like at birth and understood that within the next several months they would have to begin an arduous medical journey. Within hours of the delivery, however, the baby's grandfather—an MD himself—collared Eva. He insisted the baby be transferred to a hospital with neurosurgical capabilities. "This child needs to see a neurosurgeon immediately," he barked.

Eva was taken aback by the grandfather's insistence. Surgery was important, but it wasn't needed right away. She also knew how immensely disruptive hospital transfers were. The family would have to navigate the discharge process from one hospital, arrange transport, pack the newborn and postpartum mother in an ambulance, then start the admissions process to enter another hospital. There would be insurance issues, phone calls, evaluations. Blood tests and X-rays would be repeated. There would be new doctors and nurses to meet, a new gamut of procedures to negotiate and understand. It was an immense effort for exhausted parents who had just been through the ordeal of labor and childbirth. And it would force their focus to shift from their newborn to paperwork.

"The child will indeed need to see a neurosurgeon," Eva replied. "But it isn't necessary at this moment." She thought of the baby in the supply room, the frightened parents in the delivery room shielding their eyes. "The most important thing right now is for the parents to bond with the baby."

The grandfather stood stock-still. "He looked at me like I was a complete idiot," Eva recalled, like she'd just recommended witch doctors and garlic compresses for his grandson. But she stood her ground. She felt an immense sadness for this baby with his profound deformities, and for the parents who had so much to deal with. But it was her grief over the baby who had died in her arms in the supply closet that seemed to channel forward and dictate her actions now. This new baby would not be denied the full radiance of his parents' love. These parents would not lose this irreplaceable moment of bonding. Baby and parents deserved a protected respite before the onslaught of medical procedures that would dominate the upcoming months and years. Eva resisted the pressure and kept the baby and family where they were.

Another time, Eva was called to evaluate a newborn. This family had a regular pediatrician who would take over once the family left the hospital, but Eva was the in-house pediatrician that weekend, responsible for the baby's care for these first few days.

As she examined the baby, she noticed that the eyes were down-slanting and the ears a bit low-set. Was this Down syndrome? A rivulet of sadness scraped open inside her. Was this child going to face a lifetime of challenges? Were these parents, right now in the bliss of babyhood, about to receive crushing news? Though Down syndrome can be definitively diagnosed only with a chromosomal analysis, the pediatrician's physical exam is often the first suggestion that something might be wrong. And here the baby's eyes were down-slanting. Eva felt her soul heave a mournful sigh.

But then again, she thought, the father's eyes were a bit slanted too, so maybe it was just a family trait. She held on to the hopeful thought. The baby's ears were a bit low-set, true, but not excessively so. She examined the baby's neck. Was that the classic webbed neck that she was seeing, or was it just baby fat?

In her mind, Eva went back and forth, debating the physical features of the baby. In her soul, Eva went back and forth between sadness and optimism. Would she be delivering painful news or simply congratulating the parents on their healthy baby girl? Some features of the baby were suggestive of Down's, but they certainly weren't the textbook picture. She knew that her suspicions could easily be unfounded. The baby would need a chromosomal analysis to determine the diagnosis, but that would take some time. Eva weighed whether or not she should share her suspicions with the parents right now.

What if she was wrong, if she'd just been overly cautious during the physical exam? The parents would be saddled with horrific distress during this special bonding time—all of it unnecessary.

Maybe the whole thing could wait a few days until the family saw their pediatrician, whom they'd known for years and who would be able to spend more time with them. It would be awful to have traumatic news delivered by a doctor they barely knew who was merely doing brief early-morning rounds . . . especially if that news could be wrong.

In terms of clinical treatment, a gap of a few days would be irrelevant. There's no immediate treatment needed for Down syndrome; in fact, there's often only minor medical treatment needed at all. It is more about learning what life will be like and getting things started with speech therapy, physical therapy, family and social services. This process takes months, years. A few days wouldn't change anything.

"Back and forth I went," Eva recalled, "but since I wasn't completely sure, it seemed that it could wait a few days until they saw their own pediatrician. Why couldn't they just enjoy their little girl a little longer and fall in love? If it did turn out to be Down's, they would hear it from their own doctor. A few days wouldn't make a difference. So I said, 'Congratulations—enjoy your beautiful baby girl.'"

Eva watched the parents snuggle their baby, gazing into her eyes with the pure, unadulterated adoration a newborn evokes. It was a pristine moment, and it only comes around once. There would be time for other emotions later. Thinking again of the baby dying in the closet, Eva felt at peace with her decision to withhold her suspicions for the moment.

A week later, Eva called the pediatrician to see how things had worked out. It turned out that chromosomal testing did confirm Down syndrome. Eva felt her heart catch. Life would certainly be difficult for the child and her parents. It wasn't cancer, of course, and it wasn't Potter syndrome or even Apert syndrome, but the parents had a lot ahead of them. She felt for them, for the turbulence and confusion that they were experiencing now. It was never easy to hear that something was wrong with your child. She hoped, though, that the parents—and the baby—had benefited from those few days free of worry. A few days of pure joy, before the challenges began.

The pediatrician's voice took on a note of incredulity. "How could you have let the parents leave the hospital thinking they had a healthy baby?" she asked. The barb was unmistakable.

"But they do have a healthy baby," Eva replied, "a healthy baby who happens to have Down syndrome."

There was silence on the other end of the line.

—⚶—

Isaac Edwards was one of those patients who just grows on you. He came to my clinic because he wanted his softball-size inguinal hernia repaired, but the surgeons wouldn't operate until his blood pressure was controlled. His pressure was a sky-high 215/110 that day, despite the five medications he was taking. This was going to be a tough case, I remember thinking on that first day.

Mr. Edwards was a former heroin user but had quit drugs—and methadone—in the 1970s. He'd spent the 1980s in prison but had led a clean, quiet life since then. He was divorced before he went to prison and, during incarceration, had lost touch with his four children.

Mr. Edwards was five foot six, thin, compact, with short, cropped graying hair and a distinctive, raspy voice. "Miz Ofri," he'd always call out to me from the waiting room, his choice of appellation an endearing mix of Southern manners and Bronx casual. He was sort of a strange bird, turning up at odd times with a burning question about one of his medications or a scrawled query on a scrap of paper. He'd sometimes miss a blood test or lose a bottle of pills. Occasionally his prescriptions were stolen. Appointments were mixed up.

At first I'd pegged him as the forever-chaotic ex-addict type. But somehow he'd always manage to patch things together, even if the final result was slightly off-kilter. I grew to respect that he was, in fact, quite committed to his health and was trying hard to do the right thing.

His craggy charm appealed to me, and I was always happy to see him, even if I was frustrated that he'd forgotten to get his EKG done or had missed his appointment with the nutritionist. Mr. Edwards had this self-sufficient manner about him, though I wasn't completely confident in his ability to hold everything together. He had maintained the same address in the Bronx for some time—not necessarily a given for someone in his situation—but his phone service was intermittent, generally in tandem with whether he had a job or not.

We spent the better part of an arduous year controlling his blood pressure with an ever-changing, complex regimen of pills. I saw Mr. Edwards on a nearly monthly basis until, finally, his blood pressure eased down from the 200s to the 180s to the 160s. This was an acceptable level for surgery, and we were both ecstatic. I wrote a triumphant preoperative clearance note in the chart and sent him back to the surgery clinic to arrange for his long-awaited hernia operation.

It took several weeks to get the appointment, work out the scheduling, and make the financial arrangements, but the date for the operation was at long last set. I was so happy that we would cross this tangible line of success. We would be able to relieve him of this enormous hernia that had been troubling him for years.

But the operation never happened.

"I chickened out," Mr. Edwards told me sheepishly when he came back to my office for his next appointment.

"You what?" I was flabbergasted, given how much effort and time—on both of our parts—had gone into getting him to this surgery.

He looked down, a rueful expression on his face. "I'm afraid of needles, Miz Ofri."

"Afraid of needles?" I said, astonished. "You are probably handier with a needle than your surgeon. How can you be afraid of needles?"

He shook his head from side to side. "No needles, no way. Once you been off heroin, you can't look at no needle again. When they told me that I'd be getting an IV for the surgery . . ." He paused here, momentarily overwhelmed, it seemed, by the prospect of an IV.

I opened my mouth again to speak, but then I closed it. I realized that I had to tuck my incredulity away. This was his reality. As incongruous as it seemed to me, I had to respect it. Isaac Edwards was the one who had battled heroin and methadone. I felt for him, for what it must be like to be overpowered by a fear.

Over the next year, diabetes crept into the picture to join his hypertension. Several more pills were added to his regimen. Insulin, of course, was completely out of the question because of the needle issue. His sugar kept climbing, and I knew that we'd be facing a predicament soon.

The hypertension and diabetes were taking a toll on his kidneys, and his renal function was inching downward. Life was not going to get any easier. I was honest with Mr. Edwards and told him that dialysis was likely in the future. The nephrologist held out hope that something other than hypertension or diabetes might be affecting his kidneys, in which case there might be a treatment that could at least stave off dialysis for a few years.

But Mr. Edwards was mortally afraid of the kidney biopsy that would be needed to make such a diagnosis. "It's that needle," he said, shaking his head at his own fear. "I can't face another needle, Miz Ofri."

I told him that thrice-weekly dialysis needles would be a lot worse than a one-time biopsy and that if we could postpone dialysis for a few years it could make a real difference in his life. I pestered, pressed, and cajoled him until he finally scheduled the biopsy. But he didn't show. Three times we scheduled it, and three times he didn't show. The nephrologist gave up.

Between his hypertension, diabetes, and renal disease, the inguinal hernia—his initial medical issue—ended up on the back burner. Mr. Edwards stopped complaining about it, and I no longer examined it during our visits, since there were always acute issues that consumed our attention. One time he experienced a severe reaction to a diabetes medication, ending up hospitalized with pulmonary edema. After that, his legs swelled mercilessly, probably from his kidney disease. His blood sugar continued to plod upward, and I spent our visits talking about the necessity of insulin.

"You're wasting your breath, Miz Ofri," he'd say to me with that wry half-smile of his. "I know you a busy doc, so you ought to be saving your energy for something more productive."

But I was determined not to let his resistance sabotage his health. I was not going to let him die because of a fear of needles. Finally I achieved what I considered to be the Olympic decathlon of medical success: I introduced Mr. Edwards to an insulin pen, a newer method of delivery that didn't look like a syringe or anything remotely similar to drug paraphernalia. The needle was minuscule, and when I convinced him to try it—after I stuck the needle in my own arm—he agreed that he couldn't even feel the pinch.

It was touch-and-go at first, but after several months of cajoling and cheerleading, Mr. Edwards began taking insulin injections every night with the pen, though at a tiny, nearly placebo dose. My plan was that once I'd gotten him over the psychological hump of actually using the insulin, I'd start titrating the dose to where we'd get his sugar under control. This wouldn't reverse his kidney disease, but it could possibly slow it down and buy him time before dialysis. Success in the world of chronic disease is hard to come by, but I felt that he and I deserved a gold medal on this one.

The phone call came on a Thursday afternoon. It was my precepting day, and I was juggling a half dozen interns and residents, piles of med refills, assorted forms, and preauthorization annoyances. The woman on the phone introduced herself as a social worker from a hospital in Brooklyn. "Are you the doctor for Isaac Edwards?" she asked.

"Oh, yes," I said with a smile. "That's me . . . Miz Ofri." I signed and stamped three prescriptions while I spoke.

"I'm sorry it's taken so long to track you down," she said, "but Mr. Edwards didn't leave any next-of-kin contact or the names of any doctors."

Next of kin? The stamper slipped from my fingers. What was she talking about?

"It all happened so quickly," she said, "and there was nothing in his wallet to give us any clues. Nobody showed up to claim the body. I've been calling around all week, and finally the trail led me to you."

My stomach clenched into an iron-like knot as I realized what she was saying. "What was it?" I stammered into the phone. "Kidney failure? A heart attack? A stroke?"

She declined to give me medical details, but patched me through to a surgeon. "He was admitted on Friday with severe abdominal pain," the surgeon told me. I pulled up Mr. Edwards's chart on the computer while the surgeon spoke. I saw that he had been to our clinic just forty-eight hours earlier for a prescription refill. One of the physician assistants gave him his meds and reminded him of his appointment with me next month.

Mr. Edwards had apparently collapsed on the street from the pain and was taken by ambulance to the nearest hospital, where a CT scan revealed free air in his abdomen, an ominous sign that indicates intestinal rupture.

"We rushed him straight to the operating room," the surgeon said. "We found a knot of gangrenous intestine that was strangulated in his inguinal hernia."

That hernia! All those struggles with his blood pressure, diabetes, and renal disease, and that goddamned hernia had come back to haunt us. I could feel my body flood with rage at the horribleness, the injustice.

"We resected the dead gut, and he seemed to do well postoperatively," the surgeon continued, "but he coded the next morning, Saturday, and they couldn't bring him back. Could have been a heart attack or pulmonary embolus. We're not sure. I tried to get an autopsy, but our hospital doesn't do them anymore."

The social worker came back on the line. "We've been trying since Saturday to find a relative, even a friend. But there doesn't seem to be anyone," she said. "Our morgue can only hang on to unclaimed bodies for so long. Finally we had to send him to Potter's Field."

My anger streamed away, overcome by heartache. Potter's Field, as the cemetery is commonly called, is an isolated sliver of an island in the Long Island Sound where unclaimed New Yorkers have been interred since the Civil War. Mr. Edwards would have been buried by inmates from Rikers Island.

"Did he have any relatives that you know of?" the social worker asked me.

When I'd taken his full history at our initial meeting three years earlier, he'd told me he had been estranged from his ex-wife and four children for more than thirty years. He never came to appointments with anyone nor did he ever mention anyone in his life.

"Didn't you ever ask him," the social worker said, pressing me, "who you should call in case anything ever happened to him?"

I felt a twinge of embarrassment. It seemed obvious in retrospect, but clinic visits for a walking, talking, self-sufficient adult weren't the same as a hospital admission for a critically ill patient. Next-of-kin issues rarely came up. But, mainly, we were so busy taking care of his active medical concerns that we never got around to it. There was always his blood pressure out of control or his diabetes or the kidney biopsy or the hernia surgery that filled every visit. There were never any leftover moments for chatting about other issues. I suddenly felt terribly guilty.

I held the social worker on the phone for as long as I could as the emotional calculus took hold that this would be my last connection to Mr. Edwards. In fact, it might be the last time anyone thought about Mr. Edwards or spoke his name. After I hung up the phone, that would be it. The surgeon and the social worker would move on to other patients. Mr. Edwards would be just another case in their vast medical enterprise.

It was frightening to realize that someone could die and there might be nobody to mourn, much less reflect or even react. It dawned on me that I might have been the only person who had any regular contact with Mr. Edwards over these years. I was seized by the desire to attend his funeral, to do something to demonstrate that his life had connection. But even that wasn't possible now.

Finally I hung up the phone but continued plowing through his chart, the only palpable evidence of his life. I read and reread all the pages I'd written about him—his kidneys, his glucose, his hernia, his fear of needles—until my eyes were blurry with melancholy.

I took a deep breath and then wrote a sober expiration note in the chart, a postscript to the official documentation of his life. And then I pushed my other charts and prescriptions out of the way and wrote down everything I could remember about Mr. Edwards, suddenly desperate to solidify my recollections before they faded.

I published his story in the *New York Times*, wanting to give him some sort of formal recognition, a prayer of condolence that he deserved.[3] I used his real name in the article—Isaac Edwards—hoping against hope that someone out there would recognize him, that someone else in this world would join me in carrying a bit of him in our memories, so that Mr. Edwards wouldn't have died completely alone.

A few weeks after his death, his name popped up on my clinic roster for his appointment that had been scheduled earlier. I was unprepared for the claw that seized my gut. I stood at the front desk of the clinic staring at the name Isaac Edwards on my sheet while the buzz of the medical world swirled efficiently around me. The indifference was like salt in my wound. Couldn't anyone else see what had happened? Didn't anyone notice the exquisite sorrow of a man dying invisibly? At that moment, I felt so isolated in my grief, so heartsick at the loneliness of his death. Isaac Edwards had fallen in the forest, and no one had heard.

—⁂—

Grief tugs insistently at doctors. We form relationships—like all humans colliding in this world—but our partners in these relationships die off with a regularity that isn't common elsewhere. A thread of sorrow weaves through the daily life of medicine, even during the mundane and pedestrian encounters. It is disease, after all, that we are dealing with, not misdemeanors, philosophies, or building foundations.

At times, every patient encounter can seem like a countdown to death. Usually, our denial-of-death instinct keeps such thoughts handily buried, but not always. Whether it is the traumatic deaths that residents like Eva face, the ceaseless stream of deaths in oncology, or the singular poignant loss of a Mr. Edwards, it's a steady sapping of human reserves.

After staring at Mr. Edwards's name on the list for what seemed an eternity, I walked numbly back to my office and stood in front of the door, unable to open it. A patient was waiting inside—alive and kicking but saddled with a medley of chronic ailments, one of which would surely do him in eventually. I didn't know if I could do it again: invest and then grieve.

I wanted to sit still with the grief of Mr. Edwards. I wanted the world to stop for a few minutes to focus on the death of this man. It wasn't just that it was all still raw for me after just one month but that I felt an obligation to hold on to his memory, a duty to remember, because there was no one else to remember. I knew that the patient waiting in the room and all the future waves of patients and their unique and poignant stories would press up against my memory of Isaac Edwards. Like a balloon straining from a child's hand, his memory might escape my grasp, despite my best intentions, and steal silently, forlornly into the endless sky. And then there would be no one to recall his quirky charm, the trials and tribulations of his last few years, the irony and sadness of his demise.

I didn't want to start again—meeting someone I would likely lose, forming one more memory that might edge out that of Isaac Edwards—but of course I had to. I knew that. I recalled what a colleague once told me as I was contemplating having a second child. My first child occupied every ounce of my love and my energy, and finding emotional space for another seemed impossible. My colleague—a wise physician and a father of three—reassured me. "Your capacity simply expands," he told me. "Your heart grows bigger and there is enough room to love more."

I thought about those words as I stood before the door. In some ways, grief is an aspect of love, a reflection of the ability to connect. As the heart can grow bigger to allow more love, it can also do so for grief. I don't want any more of my patients to die, but I know that they will. And although I don't *want* more grief in my life, I know that the connections that permit grief to occur are the connections that keep us—doctors and patients—alive.

And so I closed my eyes, drew a long, angling breath, and turned the knob.

—ᴍ—

For physicians, sadness is part of the job. There is pain in watching your patients suffer; there is grief when they die. Of course, there is also joy in medicine—helping patients get well, even the muted joy of helping patients die well—but it is the sorrowful side of medicine that obviously weighs heaviest. How the sadness is handled by the physician has a powerful impact on the medical care received by the patients. If the grief is relentlessly suppressed—as in Eva's experience during residency—the result can be a numb physician who is unable to invest in a new patient. This lack of investment can lead to rote medical care—impersonal at best, shoddy at worst. At the other end of the spectrum is the doctor who is inundated with grief and can't function because of the overwhelming sorrow. Burnout is a significant risk in both these cases, and that erodes the quality of medical care.

There is no perfect formula for handling grief, no easy algorithm to teach. Integrating sadness while still being able to function and give of yourself is necessarily a work in progress. It is something akin to two coils spinning. The coil of sadness never stops—there is always an awareness that your patients are suffering and the memory of the patients you've lost. The other coil is the engine of what you are giving to your new patients, the investment in their lives and health. Though nobody desires grief in one's life, wise and experienced clinicians will tell you that they'd never want that coil to disappear. It keeps alive a necessary appreciation of medicine, of what it means to have the privilege of entering other people's lives.

Ultimately, the two coils are synergistic. The poignancy from the sadness can actually be the fuel for what flows to the next patient. But this requires both the individual physician and the surrounding medical community to be attuned to grief and to allow it its due.

Julia, part four

After Julia's hospitalization in the ICU, she had a difficult year. Daily activities became more challenging, though she was still somehow managing. There were a few other, shorter admissions to the hospital. Each time Julia came home weaker, improved a bit at home, but settled at a slightly lower notch. The descent had truly begun, for her heart and for mine.

I had been dreading this moment for years, and now it was here. Every time she mentioned her children—a birthday, a communion, a graduation—an unsparing chill would abrade the inside of my chest. It was almost too much to bear.

I realized that I simply wasn't ready to contemplate Julia's death. All these years of her good health had allowed the denial to nest within me, to the point that I had convinced myself that she would never die. I knew that her heart was doomed, but every month or two she'd appear in my clinic for an appointment, looking basically the same as at the previous visit. Year in and year out. Facts on the ground, you might call it.

It was like I'd had a long-term relationship with the healthy, robust Julia, the one who wasn't going to die, and like any creature of habit, I wasn't prepared for when the relationship changed. But as the months wore on, I could no longer delude myself. That healthy Julia was fading before my eyes, aging and weakening in real time.

The instinct in medicine to do something is a powerful one, and I found myself frantically rejiggering her medications, rechecking labs, rethinking her entire treatment regimen. I could feel the panic enrobing me, but I was determined to stay one step ahead of it. If I could just think harder, think quicker, think smarter, I could stave things off.

But I was simply rearranging deck chairs. I knew this, yet I couldn't stop myself. Julia's failing heart was an implacable force, and it was going to sink her no matter what I did. It was time to prepare.

Julia never wanted to talk about "it," but our casual conversations helped me keep tabs on the situation. Her sister Claribel was helping out with the children, taking over many of the day-to-day tasks. It was clear that she would be their eventual caretaker.

Julia also received assistance from her landlord, Ernesto, a gentle Cuban exile who'd taken his Guatemalan tenants under his wing. He helped out with whatever physical tasks came up so that Julia wouldn't have to overexert herself. He even spotted her on the rent a few times when cash was in short supply. Julia's children grew to see Ernesto as another uncle in the family.

This web of connections reassured me that Julia would not be alone when things worsened and that Lucita and Vasco would be cared for with love when the time came. But it was the idea that the time would come, that there would be a time *after*, a time without Julia, that I just could not reconcile myself to.

There is a concept called anticipatory grief, in which a person grieves before the actual event has taken place—before the death, before the divorce, before the job loss. Some psychologists view this as a way for a person to orient herself to the impending loss, to "rehearse" the emotions that will be experienced. For some people, it is a way to sort out unresolved issues and begin to think about closure.

But I wasn't having any of it. Not one stinking drop! The grief—when it came—would be awful enough. I didn't need to jump-start my misery. And so, biting back the tears that I refused to allow, I watched my precious Julia waning before me, day by day.

CHAPTER 5

Burning with Shame

Precisely two weeks after completing internship, I proceeded to nearly kill a patient. July marked the start of my second year of residency at Bellevue Hospital, and it was my first time being fully in charge of a patient.

My patient arrived in florid DKA—diabetic ketoacidosis—a life-threatening condition in which lack of insulin causes metabolic cataclysm. It was a classic Bellevue DKA story: arrested during a smalltime drug deal, tossed into an NYPD holding cell, unable to access his insulin. The patient sat around as his sugar wormed its way to stratospheric levels. When he began to vomit and slur his speech, the police brought him to the ER.

We were situated in a cramped, dingy corner of the old Bellevue ER next to the trauma slot. There was a single narrow desk overflowing with X-rays, charts, coffee cups, stethoscopes, and the glutei maximi of staff who perched there trying to conduct medical business while paramedics wheeled in shotgun wounds and motor vehicle accidents.

With my intern looking to me for guidance—he, with the ink still wet on his MD diploma, and me, with a scant single year more experience—I placed the patient on an intravenous insulin drip. DKA is one of those rare, gratifying conditions in which a patient arrives in extremis and, with the deft handling of insulin, is readily cured. I felt a surge of pride as we watched our patient gain consciousness, get cranky, and then demand double meal portions.

Our patient's glucose returned to normal. With palpable triumph, I handed a "d/c insulin drip" order to the nurse. I was officially declaring our patient cured.

The nurse took the order from me while passing a bottle of saline to another medical resident. "Do you want to give an injection of long-acting insulin before stopping the drip?" she asked me as the clerk pressed two more charts in her direction.

I thought for a moment. Why would I want to use the sledge-hammer of long-acting insulin after eight hours of our meticulous adjustments with the insulin drip? "No," I said, turning to my intern, capitalizing on the teaching moment. "If we push him overboard with long-acting insulin, it'll be stuck in his system for hours, and his sugar could bottom out. Let's just keep checking his glucose hourly and give him short-acting insulin as needed."

The nurse raised her eyebrows ever so slightly.

The intern nodded with me—my logic was obvious. The nurse shrugged and went back to her work.

My logic was indeed obvious. It was also wrong. Right-out-of-the-textbook wrong. The very thing you are *supposed* to do in DKA is administer long-acting insulin just before stopping the drip, otherwise the patient will turn right around and slide back into DKA, which is what our patient gamely proceeded to do.

When the blood tests revealed dangerously rising potassium and acid pH, I called the senior resident for help.

My intern and I stood nervously while the senior resident scrutinized the numbers. She wrinkled her brow for perhaps three seconds, then shot me a withering look. "Didn't you give him long-acting insulin before you turned off the drip?" she demanded. "A little longer like this and he'll be comatose! Next thing you know we'll be calling a code."

I tried to describe our methodical treatment and how logic would dictate—wouldn't it?—that we shouldn't muck up a tenuous situation with long-acting medications, that we wouldn't want to harm the patient by pushing his sugar too low, that we . . .

My words began to run up against each other, progressively garbling under the weight of her granite stare until they petered out into silence. Another trauma case had just been wheeled in and surgeons bustled past us shouting competing orders.

"What were you thinking?" the senior resident said, her normally pleasant voice now like a drill sergeant's.

I stood there stone still as my brain cells slowly dissolved into muck.

"What *were* you thinking?" she repeated, her voice now thundering through the ER, despite the pandemonium swelling around us. Lives were at stake left and right, and she clearly wasn't going to let me get out of this.

I couldn't even muster a whisper, knowing that my intern, who had nodded so trustingly at my earlier pronouncements, was standing not four inches from me. Scrub-clad bodies were jostling against me in the cramped space of the ER, but I felt a gulf widen around me, as though I'd just lost control of my bladder and was standing in an ever-growing puddle of mortification. My cognitive functions ground to a halt, and for the life of me I could not produce a monosyllabic response, much less an intelligent explanation.

What *had* I been thinking?

Had I simply forgotten the part about the long-acting insulin? Had I misread the textbook? Had I slept through the lecture on DKA? Was I just not smart enough to be a doctor?

The senior resident stared at me, waiting for an answer. I knew I'd made a mistake, but this prolonged agony—thirty seconds clawed out to an eon—was not helping me know that awful truth any better.

If only my intern weren't standing right next to me. Alone I could probably have handled the rightful reprimand, but the humiliation in his presence was unbearable.

The senior resident wrenched the pen from my hand and furiously wrote stat orders to restart the insulin drip and to administer a shot of long-acting insulin along with a dose of calcium and bicarbonate to avoid cardiac arrest from the dangerously skewed potassium and pH. For a moment I thought she was going to wrench the patient out of my hands as well.

When she finally departed, I couldn't even raise my eyes to my intern. All I wanted to do was crawl under a rock and weep. But I couldn't. There was an intern waiting for guidance, and a patient who needed medical care.

"Let's, uh, check the patient's fluid status," I stammered, the heat in my cheeks making it difficult to articulate words, "and then draw another set of labs."

"Got it," the intern said. Matter-of-factly, he began tearing open gauze pads, pulling out alcohol swabs, labeling test tubes. It was the normalcy of his actions that allowed me to breathe again. The absolute ordinariness of his conduct was an act of compassion that I've never forgotten. His spark of humanity permitted me to regroup, and we returned to our patient, whom we were able to—once again—rescue from the throes of DKA. In two days he was back with the cops.

The senior resident graduated and went off to another job. The intern became a fine doctor in private practice. I continued an academic career at Bellevue. Since that day, I have never in my life failed to inject long-acting insulin before stopping an insulin drip.

Lesson learned. Doctor reeducated; mistake never to be made again.

Patient did fine, suffered no ill effects. Near-miss caught in time by the system of supervision by more experienced doctors.

Case closed.

But should it have been?

Certainly in those days, that's how such near-misses and errors were treated. If this had happened today, there might be a different ending to the story. If I had been a medical resident in today's world, the patient would have been approached by the medical team and possibly by risk management, informed of a medical error that had potentially been life-threatening (despite its being near-miss in terms of outcome), and given an apology; he would be told that the hospital and doctor accepted full responsibility.

This new approach, commonly referred to as a full-disclosure policy, started as a way to rein in the spiraling malpractice suits that hospitals were facing. But it was also recognized that it was simply the right thing to do, that an acknowledgment and apology could be meaningful to the patient—and perhaps even the doctor—trying to recover from the trauma of a medical error.

As a more mature physician now, I can accept this as the ethical thing to do. But as a fledgling doctor, already humiliated down to the calluses on my feet, I couldn't imagine anything more dreadful. I'd sooner have accepted ten rounds on that carnival ride where you're thrown back against the wall of the barrel while the floor repeatedly plummets from under you.

Taking responsibility wasn't the hard part—I'd already done that. I spent weeks afterward flagellating my brain for its incompetence, berating myself for my idiocy. But the idea of dragging my sorry self into the patient's room, looking him straight in the eye, and explaining that I had committed a grave error because of my incompetence—one that had threatened his life, kept him in the ICU for an extra day, exposed him to another day's worth of ICU pathogens and procedural risks, not to mention costs—was humiliating beyond comprehension.

It seems entirely obvious: doctors need to apologize for their errors, even if the patients got lucky and did not suffer irreparable harm. But in the real world of medicine, doctors have notorious difficulty with apology (even beyond the fear-of-lawsuits issue).

A few years ago I stumbled across the book *On Apology*[1] by Aaron Lazare, a psychiatrist and former dean of University of Massachusetts School of Medicine. It was a revelation, not just about medicine, but about human interaction in general.

Lazare discusses three distinct emotions that influence the decision to apologize: empathy, guilt, and shame. Empathy—the ability to identify with someone else's suffering—is certainly a prerequisite for a genuine apology.

But then Lazare distinguishes carefully between guilt and shame. Guilt is usually associated with a particular incident and can dissipate when the issue is resolved. But shame reflects a failure of one's entire being. While guilt often prods a person to make amends, shame induces a desire to hide.

Shame, Lazare writes, is "an emotional reaction to the experience of failing to live up to one's image of oneself." Here, I believe, he puts his finger on the precise fiber of resistance in doctors.

When I think back to that moment in the emergency room when the senior resident berated me for my error, it was not guilt but shame that overpowered me. Of course I felt guilty—that was the easy part. I had no trouble with berating myself for the error. But it was the shame that was paralyzing. It was the shame of realizing that I was not who I thought I was, that I was not who I'd been telling my patient and my intern I was. It wasn't that I was forgetful or momentarily distracted. It was not that I was neglectful or even uncaring. It was that up until that moment, I'd thought I was a competent, even excellent, doctor. In one crashing moment of realization, that persona shattered to bits.

One could argue that this is a rather self-centered way of viewing the entire episode: how the doctor felt. After all, it was the patient who experienced the error. But it is precisely the doctor's emotion—particularly shame—that stands as the major impediment to the full-disclosure policies that are increasingly demanded. Even if evidence convincingly demonstrates that disclosure and apology lead to fewer lawsuits, the desired culture of openness will come about only when we address the issue of shame. No matter how rational we doctors claim to be, the fragility of the human heart can prevail over data, ethics, even laws.

One has to wonder, then, why it is that doctors feel their entire sense of self at risk when they admit errors. Perhaps it is the culture of perfection in medicine that fosters a strictly binary analysis: either you are an excellent doctor or you are a failure.

In 1953, the British pediatrician and psychoanalyst Donald Winnicott introduced the idea of the "good enough" mother.[2] This was, and still is, a revolutionary concept. Parents often bend over backward to achieve perfection in meeting their child's every need. Winnicott argued that this wasn't necessary, that good enough was, well, good enough. (He actually stressed that good enough might even be better than perfection in that it fosters children's healthy adaptation to the realities of human interaction.)

In most aspects of life, we seem able to accept this and deal satisfactorily with the good-enough teacher, the good-enough accountant, the good-enough plumber. But there is no room for the good-enough doctor. An error redounds not as a misstep that can be remedied with education but as an intrinsic incrimination of one's very being . . . not to mention a dead or gravely injured patient.

Shame worms its way into the heart and is remembered like few other things. I'll admit that the intricacies of DKA physiology have grown a bit fuzzy over the years. But the details of my insulin error in the dingy Bellevue ER are crisply stored in the linings of my heart. To this day, when I teach my students about DKA, I emphasize that clinical point with the vehemence of Moses on Sinai: "Thou shalt not turn off the insulin drip until long-acting insulin hath been administered."

Because shame is so global and its consequences so devastating, human beings automatically erect walls to hide their shame, making it one of the most challenging emotions to examine, much less confront. This makes intuitive sense because the sine qua non of shame is discovery of a flaw and the attendant fear in anticipation of its exposure. Hiding and covering up are intrinsic to shame.

People often use the phrase "I was mortified" to describe their shame. The word *mortify* suggests, etymologically, that we can die from our shame. Indeed, at that moment in the ER, being screamed at by my resident, I could almost feel myself dying away on the spot. In fact, for many endless minutes, that seemed preferable. Not in the literal sense, of course, but I wanted to evaporate, to disappear, to expire from that horrific moment of shame. The very last thing I could envision was owning up to my error to the patient.

I sometimes wonder whether doctors are more shame-prone than most people, or whether the medical profession itself is more shame-prone than other professions, though shame is, of course, a universal emotion. Given that we do not accept the idea of the good-enough doctor, that physicians are always striving for and expecting perfection, every doctor feels that he or she falls short to some degree. Perhaps shame and self-blame are built into the system because of an unrealistic and pervasive expectation of perfection.

In-depth interviews with doctors who have been part of a medical error demonstrate a strong propensity for self-blame, with the attendant shame.[3] When talking about components of an error that could be attributed to the system or to others, the doctor will use distant and impersonal language, such as "The fracture was missed on the initial X-ray." But when the doctor is directly involved, the language turns bluntly inward: "I missed the early signs of bleeding. My patient died because of my mistake. This will haunt me forever."

Stereotype suggests that doctors lean toward blaming others or the system for mistakes. This set of interviews suggests otherwise, that doctors overwhelmingly direct blame inward. This may reflect an overinflated sense of power, that doctors feel they have the innate capability to effect change. Outcomes—whether good or bad—are attributed to personal actions. So when an error does happen, doctors may more easily indict themselves than recognize the shortcomings of their profession as a whole. This preserves their sense of what doctors are capable of.

The current attempts to decrease medical error focus on systems issues—pre-op checklists, no look-alike medication bottles, computerized ordering to replace handwritten prescriptions, surgery sites marked directly on the patient's body before the operation, computerized algorithms for everything from urinary catheters to blood thinners. Based on the current research on the causes of error, the systems approach should offer the highest yield in reducing preventable error, and hospitals are rightly investing resources in this area.

This approach, however, may have some unintended consequences. Physicians might (unconsciously) find this threatening to their fundamental beliefs about their tribe and the profession of medicine. This is not to say that these systems issues should not be broached, but that there might be resistance because of this underlying psychology. Certainly many doctors are chafing against the increasing pressure to use clinical algorithms to treat many common conditions such as pneumonia and urinary infections. Administrators see these algorithms as a definite plus, since it standardizes care and offers tangible benchmarks to measure quality (more on that later). Doctors, however, see it as a threat to their independence, an insulting regression to cookbook medicine. They feel that their professional skills and their clinical judgment for individual patients supersede rote recipes. They want to be in charge, which also means taking the blame at times.

Self-blame is, of course, not completely bad. Recognizing a personal role in an error can cause many doctors to redouble their commitments to being responsible and knowledgeable clinicians. "You learn by mistakes," one doctor interviewed in the study said. "Unfortunately they are real mistakes and there are real consequences, but you can't ruminate over each mistake forever. You internalize it and it makes you a more careful physician, a better doctor."[4]

The question therefore seems to be: Can there be appropriate blame—that is, acknowledgment and acceptance of responsibility—without the paralyzing and counterproductive shame?

Medical students are particularly prone to this overwhelming experience of shame.[5] Being naïve and inadequately skilled when all those around you are busy saving lives is potently shameful, and unique to the field of medicine. As the lowest on the totem pole, many students feel forced to endure and even be party to imprudent things that senior doctors do. One student on rounds with a superior who made rude comments to patients commented that "all this I am part of. I would like to run back to the patients and explain." Another said, "I was ashamed because I thought the [patient] associated me with the doctor; I took the blame for his nastiness."

Interestingly, many medical students found that they identified more with patients than with other members of the team. Despite wearing the white coats of the profession, they felt like outsiders in this world, similar to the feelings of many patients. The humiliations that patients endured resonated profoundly with the students. "We have to ask our patients to undress and touch them in a way that they would never allow any other human being to do." Students observed doctors speaking callously to patients about sensitive subjects. Many of the diagnostic tests and treatments seemed to sap patients of their individuality and personhood. The students were ashamed to be part of a system that inflicted such indignities.

Shame is so potent that it prevents doctors from coming forward with a medical error, a situation that has direct implications for patient care. Of course, most doctors are not aware of the under-lying emotions that are influencing their behavior; they are simply reacting to their instincts, which often tell them that it's better to let sleeping dogs lie and just get on with the job. The sleeping dogs, though, have the potential to wake up, and the patient might be the one who gets bitten.

In *On Apology*, Aaron Lazare summarizes the personality traits common among people who have difficulty owning up and apolo-gizing: "They need to be in firm control of interpersonal situations. They need to be in control of their emotions. They need to feel right or morally superior most of the time; they believe they rarely make mistakes. They assume the world is hostile and that relationships are inherently dangerous."[6]

I might have rephrased that last sentence to read: "They assume the world is *litigious* and that *doctor-patient relationships* inherently carry a threat of lawsuit." But otherwise this sounds like an ac-curate description of many of the people with whom I attended medical school.

Lazare's description of people who are more comfortable making apologies, by contrast, includes the following insight: "When they apologize, they are merely admitting they made a mistake. Such an admission is not a threat so long as they feel good about themselves and feel that *they* are not a mistake." Doctors, it seems, have trouble making this distinction.

The field of medicine selects for and reinforces certain personal-ity traits. Despite efforts to diversify the pool of medical students by reaching into the fields of humanities and recruiting more women and minorities, the admissions process is still most successfully navi-gated by students who are driven, perfectionist, and accustomed to being at the top of the class. The cultural indoctrination of medi-cal training serves to reinforce the maladaptive characteristics that Lazare describes among those who aren't comfortable apologizing.

An intern doesn't even have to be privy to an actual lawsuit to assimilate a fear of disclosing errors. She has only to attend an old-fashioned M & M (Morbidity and Mortality) conference to see the bitter trial by peers that a resident experiences once an error comes to light. A student doesn't have to be shamed himself; seeing someone else shamed is sufficient.

When I was a third-year medical student, there was a patient on our ward with leukemia that had spread to her central nervous system. The patient was to receive two types of chemotherapy, one administered into a regular IV in the arm, and the other administered intrathecally—directly into the spinal cord sac. The patient was resting in her bed, and the heme-onc fellow was working at her bedside, preparing to administer the chemotherapy. The heme-onc fellow was a young man who hailed from one of the southern European countries. A thick mop of black hair rested on the edges of his wire-rimmed glasses. He was the quiet, hard-working type, not a man of many words. But he was known as a solid, reliable physician, and he was tolerant of a random third-year medical student tagging along to observe chemotherapy.

On the patient's bedside table sat two 10 cc syringes, each with one of the chemotherapy agents inside. The heme-onc fellow prepped the IV ports, cleaned everything with alcohol, and then donned a clean set of gloves. He grasped the intrathecal port in his right hand and then leaned over to murmur something to the patient. I couldn't make out what he'd said—I was trying my best to stay out of the way, so I'd parked myself by the foot of the bed—but the patient nodded and flashed a brave smile.

The fellow reached out his left hand for one of the syringes, then attached it to the intrathecal port. With an unfaltering grip and seemingly infinite patience, he discharged the contents of the syringe bit by bit, with none of the rambunctious cowboy moves I'd seen in other fellows. His eyes darted back and forth from the syringe to his watch and back again, timing the administration meticulously. His eyes reminded me of the metronome that had sat atop my childhood piano, steadily traversing its arc from one pole to the other.

And then, abruptly, that metronome seized up. His eyes had just departed the intrathecal port for their regularly scheduled round to the watch, but then they suddenly raced back to the syringe and fixed there. I saw his pupils widen and his face blanch. His eyes then whipped back to the port and immediately rebounded to the syringe.

There was a moment of frozen shock on his face and then he yanked the syringe out with such force that I jumped back involuntarily. "Go get the nurse," he barked to me, and I sprinted down the hall with the fear of God in me. I didn't know what had happened but I knew that it wasn't good.

Lowly medical student that I was, I was of course elbowed out of the patient's room by the subsequent deluge of nurses and other doctors. But from the urgent whispers, I pieced together that the fellow had accidentally administered the chemotherapy intended for the IV into the spinal cord sac, directly up against the neural tissues. The medical teams flew into action, but it was too late—the toxic medication had already flooded the cerebrospinal fluid.

The patient was rushed to the ICU, and she died within a week.

As a student, I couldn't gauge how much the incorrect chemotherapy versus the end-stage leukemia itself contributed to the patient's death. But what I did witness was the effect on the heme-onc fellow. From that day onward, his head seemed to be sunk forever toward the ground. I secretly watched the fellow in the weeks that followed, peering at him in the elevators and from across the hospital lobby. I don't think I ever saw him standing straight again. His posture of shame and remorse was indelible to me as a neophyte on the wards, already traumatized by witnessing a major medical error, a patient's tragic death, and now a seemingly permanently scarred doctor.

My heart broke every time I passed him in the hallway. I wished there were something I could do to somehow reach out and let him know that someone at least noticed how he was feeling. But who was I? Some invisible third-year medical student, less than nobody in the grand clinical scheme of hospital.

His error was a simple mix-up (not like my flat-out error of deciding not to give long-acting insulin to the DKA patient). His was a simple grabbing of the wrong syringe, nothing that could legitimately impugn his intellect, his abilities, his dedication. But the error, even though entirely inadvertent, resulted in terrible harm. One random event culminated in a patient's death and a physician's evident searing pain. Neither could be undone.

I've often wondered whether the heme-onc fellow was ever able to regain his footing after the episode. Were there compassionate teachers and colleagues who tried to ease his suffering? Did he ever connect with the patient's family to acknowledge the error and try to assuage their suffering? Did he go on to become an oncologist, helping legions of patients through their most difficult illnesses? Or was he frightened off from clinical medicine because of this, perhaps choosing research or administration—some aspect of medicine that didn't involve patients' lives and the possibility of harming them? Or maybe he quit medicine altogether and sequestered himself in some office job where the worst harm he could inflict was flubbing paperwork.

All medical training programs now include education about medical error. M & M conferences have been largely shorn of their accusatory histrionics and are now rightly geared toward helping doctors learn from errors. But there is always the issue of blame—even if unspoken—and of course the attendant humiliation and shame. The lesson absorbed by medical trainees is multifold: I'd better do my damnedest to be a good, smart doctor. I've got to be careful not to make mistakes or hurt anyone. And if a mistake happens, I sure as hell better not tell anyone.

Rarely is the issue of shame addressed. It seems out of the realm of medical education—fodder only for those on the couch with their analysts. But it is the elephant in the room. No doctor will easily fess up to error when a core sense of self is at risk. It's difficult to develop policy that addresses such a murky and uncomfortable issue as shame. But it wouldn't hurt for the senior faculty—the chairs, the division chiefs, the master clinicians—to talk publicly to trainees about their own errors and specifically address how they dealt with the shame. The very fact of these doctors continuing to be doctors—highly successful ones—despite their errors and the accompanying assaults on their self-definition would itself be a potent lesson to the students and interns. It *is* possible to hold one's head up after an error, to admit that errors are part and parcel of human existence, even in medicine. It is possible to see the error as an aspect of oneself, not the defining characteristic of oneself.

Medical error is rarely as cut-and-dried as what happened with the heme-onc fellow who picked up one syringe instead of another. More often it is an issue of degree, or judgment, or timing, or communication, something much more of a shade of gray. Yet most doctors internalize these errors as black-and-white, convinced of a direct causality from their actions to a bad outcome. This dovetails with the conclusions of the interviews with doctors about errors, mentioned earlier in this chapter.[7] Doctors have a strong sense—perhaps an overinflated sense—of the effects of their individual actions. This can reinforce their sense of professionalism and their duty toward their patients, but it also leaves them vulnerable to profound and lasting scars when things don't go well.

The shame that redounds from these errors does nothing to make these doctors better clinicians or improve patient care. In fact, it usually has the opposite effect. A group of researchers in New Zealand[8] explored this phenomenon by examining the short-term and long-term reactions of doctors against whom patients had filed disciplinary complaints (which included accusations of medical errors and as well as other patient concerns). Two-thirds of the doctors felt angry and depressed in the days and weeks after receiving the disciplinary complaint. One-third felt guilty and ashamed. One-third lost all joy and pleasure in the practice of medicine. The shame component lingered, sometimes for years. Doctors retained strong emotional responses long after the incident—anger, depression, cynicism, wariness toward patients.

A classic study of medical error polled more than 250 medical residents who had each committed a serious medical error, the type that led to severe adverse outcomes or even death.[9] Only half of the residents ever discussed the error with their attendings, and only a quarter talked with the patients and families. But this minority who discussed the errors and accepted responsibility for them were much more likely to have made constructive changes in their behavior to help prevent future errors.

These findings reinforce the idea that creating an atmosphere that is conducive to doctors stepping forward with their medical errors is critically important. The shame that surrounds error keeps mistakes and near-misses hidden. The doctors suffer, but current and future patients bear the heaviest brunt.

—〰—

Many years after my DKA incident, I ran into that senior resident; I had not seen her since our training. Ironically, perhaps prophetically, we were brought together not in the fellowship of doctorhood, but in the fellowship of patienthood. We found each other, both hulkingly pregnant, in the waiting room of an obstetrician's office. We chatted easily about jobs, spouses, families, career milestones.

As the pleasant words of long-lost colleagues circled politely around us, all I could see were the grimy, greenish walls of the Bellevue ER just behind her head, which is where I stared during that dressing-down she'd given me so many years ago. I doubted if she even remembered that incident. But for me, the shame of my error and the resultant loss of self-esteem would not release their grip on my soul. Although our meeting now was a joyous one—colleagues reconnecting, the shared excitement of new lives about to begin—I couldn't keep away the torment of that long-ago day. I couldn't even bring myself to mention the episode, even though she might have offered belated words that could have eased my lingering shame. Instead, I sat through the ultrasound of my first baby silently revisiting the details of how I'd nearly killed a patient.

Ultimately, it took almost twenty years before I could write about what happened that day in the emergency room.[10] Despite being a senior faculty member, well established now in my field, I found it extraordinarily difficult to put those words to paper. Dissecting the moment, turning out the layers of shame into the bright light, was a palpable agony. But the very palpableness of it was somehow therapeutic.

The drawing forth of those emotions—which resisted mightily!—was exhausting. But in the same way that an intense physical exertion exhausts but also somehow fortifies, I felt different afterward. There was no magical resolution. The ache surely remains, but writing gave me the chance to scrabble about in the mud with the emotions and arrive at a stalemate of sorts.

Lord knows I will never take DKA for granted. If so much as a single cc of an insulin drip is running into the veins of one of my patients, I am hovering like a hawk, compulsively checking and re-checking every minutia of lab data. But even more, I will never take the experience of shame for granted. As my senses are now forever alert for the slightest hint of ketoacidosis, they are also alert for the slightest hints of shame.

If I witness a situation in which a doctor, or nurse, or patient is somehow being shamed, I now jump in to deflect or assuage. Being a bystander is no longer an option. Preventing even one case of unnec-essary shame and humiliation will have as much ultimate beneficial effect—at least I hope—as injecting long-acting insulin before the drip is turned off.

Bringing down the rate of medical error requires work on many fronts—from hospital systems to medication labeling to communi-cation technology. Laws that offer some protection for doctors who disclose errors to patients and offer apologies are beginning to crop up, though it's not yet clear whether they will truly decrease lawsuits and certainly not clear that they will offer any protection to doctors from the harms of shame.[11]

But at the most basic level, doctors need to be able to come for-ward with their errors and near-misses, otherwise we will never know where the problems lay. Easing the legal landscape for disclosure is necessary but not nearly sufficient to foster openness about medical errors. Emotions cannot be legislated away. It is our inner landscapes that need to be tended to. Unless we can somehow defuse the shame and loss of self-definition that accompany the admission of medical errors, the gut instinct to hide an error will always be the first lynx to pounce upon the heart.

Julia, part five

City hospitals have a reputation for plenty of unappetizing characteristics—chaos, inefficiency, poor resources, difficult patients, jaded staff. Bellevue, as the oldest public hospital in the United States, is not immune to these challenges. Since 1736, it has been serving the downtrodden of New York City and has entered the public imagination as the hospital for crazies. It certainly does have those—what with more than three hundred psychiatry beds and two entire wards just for Rikers Island prisoners.

But these iconic stereotypes overshadow the immense superlatives of Bellevue. It's the designated receiving hospital for the president of the United States should something occur while he (or she) visits New York City. It's the hospital of choice for New York City's police and fire departments. It has world-class trauma, microsurgery, and emergency services. When limbs get severed during construction accidents, the ambulance brings the patient to Bellevue. It has the resources and skills to handle bioterrorism and epidemics. Bellevue excels in treating survivors of torture, patients with substance abuse, and children with psychiatric illnesses. It has the know-how and multilingualism to offer the most hospitable environment for immigrants from all over.

The thing that is most obscured by the negative stereotypes, however, is that Bellevue has heart, in bounteous supply. The overwhelming majority of people who work at Bellevue care deeply about their patients and specifically choose to work in a city hospital because of a commitment to this population. I've witnessed countless examples of staff going the extra mile for patients to help them find anything from clean socks to Ghanaian *egusi* stew to plane tickets to Chiapas.

But nothing in my decades at Bellevue prepared me for the forces set into motion when Julia tipped off that Starling curve. Her case had come to the attention of the medical director of the hospital, who himself was fluent in Spanish and passionate about immigrant issues. A team of social workers, nurses, and doctors assembled, determined to save Julia.

It's hard to say precisely what it was about Julia that galvanized such dedication. Her sweet, unassuming personality certainly brought out the best in everyone. But there were lots of patients at Bellevue with lovely personalities. Perhaps it was the starkness of her case, the seeming injustice of it on a humanitarian level. Or perhaps it was her life story, which she shared gradually as she opened up to the team.

Julia was born in a tiny rural village, barely even on the map of Guatemala. Her parents were subsistence farmers who struggled to provide for their family. But both external and internal forces made this a formidable challenge. Externally, it was the utter collapse of Guatemalan society due to civil war, corruption, and drugs. There was no end to murders, anarchy, and violence.

Internally, Julia's family suffered more than its fair share of calamity. One brother died of a brain tumor; one sister of ovarian cancer; another sister of heart failure. Two more siblings faced ovarian cancer and heart failure, but survived with treatment. And those were just the medical calamities. One sister suffered vicious domestic violence. Julia's first husband was kidnapped, and Julia was left with nothing but a severed hand on her doorstep.

Julia, who had never left her village her entire life, finally decided it was time to escape. She needed a better life for herself, and for her son Vasco, who'd never fully recovered from his meningitis in infanthood. Her trip to America, however, was a descent into hell beyond anything she'd experienced in Guatemala. The coyotes sold her into prostitution, and she was gang-raped on a daily basis. In the end, she was dumped at the side of a road. That she survived and somehow made it to New York astounded me, and apparently everyone else.

That she retained her gentle, sweet nature was a testament to an internal spirit we could hardly conceive of.

Bellevue closed ranks around Julia, determined to move mountains to get her a heart. The logistical, financial, and legal issues were immense. From the top of the hospital hierarchy to the bottom, people called in their chips, contacting friends, lawyers, reporters, transplant hospitals, politicians, anyone who might help.

Late in the summer, Julia married Ernesto, her landlord who'd been a protective neighbor from the start. Beyond his generous and loving nature, Ernesto possessed something else, something that Cubans have in greater supply than any other Latino immigrant groups: citizenship.

Bellevue's social workers sprang into action, processing Julia's papers to apply for a green card and Medicaid. The cardiology team pressed her case to the transplant centers. The hospital administration expedited the myriad of pre-transplant preparations. And then Columbia University accepted her into their transplant program. She was, after all, the perfect candidate.

The impossible had been achieved: Julia was on the list!

It was as though a yoke had been unhitched from my body and the tense coils of tamped-down grief snapped open. I knew that being on the list was no guarantee of getting a heart. Matches were tough to find and hundreds of patients died while waiting. But at long last we finally had a chance.

I took a full breath for what seemed like the first time in months, and it came in like a cool rush of rainwater—clean, silvery, relieving. Julia was on the list!

CHAPTER 6

Drowning

There was no question that Joanne would become a doctor—not in her mind, and not in anyone else's mind. Both of her parents and grandfathers were doctors, as were an uncle and two cousins. Even her maternal grandmother was a doctor; she had attended medical school in the 1920s and was one of only two women in her graduating class. Medicine was just what Joanne's family did.

Joanne had entertained thoughts of becoming an architect, but that simply wasn't an option in this family tree. Her father said that she could always change her mind once she'd finished medical school, but it was clear that he couldn't imagine how anyone would not love medicine once that threshold was crossed.

Like her two brothers, Joanne trundled off to medical school after college, though she was younger than most of her classmates. With her sharp mind and her father's encouragements, Joanne had graduated high school at fifteen and completed her undergraduate degree at nineteen at a women's college near her home. The medical school she attended in Philadelphia was the last medical school in America to have gone co-ed—and there weren't many co-eds there yet—so there was quite a bit that was new for her.

And yet, there was much that was familiar. Like other students who came from families steeped in the medical profession, Joanne already possessed a cultural framework for the field. Like a child brought up in a bilingual home, she had an instinctiveness for settling into the medical world, unlike students such as Curtis Climer, who were becoming the first doctors in their families. These students were like the greenhorns on Ellis Island—dazed and disoriented in the glare of the new world.

The first two years of medical school—the classroom years—were intellectually stimulating. It was exciting to learn what everyone else in her family knew. But what most defined her first two years of medical school was starting her own family.

Joanne had met Robert while she was still in college. They were already dating when she entered medical school. Robert was handsome, smart, and confident, clear that he was going to become a surgeon. Although he was one year older than Joanne, he entered medical school one year behind her, because of her academic acceleration.

They were married at the end of Joanne's first year of medical school. Six months later, they were both surprised when Joanne became pregnant. They hadn't planned on having a baby so soon, but here it was. Joanne came to take it in stride, as simply the way life was turning out, but Robert was not so sanguine. This was not what he wanted—not now, at least, not when he was just getting started in his medical training.

The third year of medical school—the meat of the clinical years—was an oddly exhilarating time for Joanne. She was finally out of the classroom, on the wards, and discovering the thrill of clinical medicine. "I'm a people person," she said, "and I loved the chance to talk to patients." This was when she really understood why her relatives had all become doctors—it was fascinating, stimulating, and it even seemed you could do some good at the same time. Jeremy was born in the middle of all this clinical excitement. So on top of learning how to insert IVs, put in sutures, and read CT scans, she had to juggle midnight feedings, changing diapers, and of course facing the ever-present challenge of babysitter coverage.

Nevertheless, Joanne managed to incorporate these strands of her life, hitting her stride in both medicine and mothering. Robert, however, found this unanticipated foray into parenthood unsettling and gradually began to distance himself. He seemed to wish that the baby had never arrived, or if it had to, that there would be a traditional wife/mother staying home with it.

Joanne began to suspect that perhaps Robert wanted to be *the* doctor in the family and felt competitive with Joanne (who was always one step ahead of him in training). Joanne had initially seen Robert as confident, cool, and together, but now these traits were starting to feel like arrogance. The stereotype of the surgery personality was coming to the fore.

Joanne chose to do rehabilitation medicine for her residency, figuring that this would offer relatively stable hours. After all, if Robert was going to have the demanding schedule of a surgery resident, then, for the sake of Jeremy and any future children, at least one parent had to have reliable hours.

But two things happened during her residency. The first was that she found rehab medicine to be boring and depressing. Her main caseload was young men with spinal-cord injuries from gunshot wounds who were never going to get better. She found herself longing for the excitement of real medicine, where things happened, where you could actually help patients. The second thing was that Robert bailed out.

Now Joanne was a single mother working in a field she hated. After two years in rehab medicine, she realized that this was untenable and switched to emergency medicine. The excitement was palpable—treating trauma victims, overdoses, heart attacks, acute strokes. It was so much fun that she didn't even mind repeating internship. She was gaining the skills to handle anything at a moment's notice, and this knowledge made her feel accomplished.

But the work was tiring, as was parenting a toddler. After finishing a full day in the emergency room and then coming home to care for Jeremy, she would be absolutely drained. She would drop onto the couch with a glass of wine after getting Jeremy to sleep, amazed that she had made it through the day. Her emergency medicine residency lasted three grueling years.

One day, during her final month of residency, her attending sat back in his chair and said, "The ER is yours. I'll be here in case you need me, but you run the show." It was a huge job, running an entire emergency room, but Joanne found that she was able to do it and do it well. Even while raising a preschooler singlehandedly.

"It all clicked," she said. "I knew that this was what I wanted to do, and that I was capable of doing it." Joanne had officially joined her family's medical lineage.

She went to work in an urban emergency room in downtown Philadelphia in the late 1980s and early 1990s. These years coincided with the peak years of the crack and PCP epidemic—which took a toll on emergency rooms nationwide, with its exceptional violence, crack-induced psychosis, and generalized mayhem. It was also the turbulent early years of AIDS, before the powerful antiretroviral medications turned AIDS into a manageable chronic illness.

Crack, PCP, and AIDS certainly added to the stress of her days, but, ironically, what wore down Joanne the most was that ER medicine turned out to be—in her concise summary—"the same shit over and over again." Once she got beyond the excitement of mastering most of the basic clinical scenarios during residency, everything began to feel repetitive. And worse, so much of ER medicine appeared to be the fallout of patients not taking care of themselves.

A cardiac patient would be lackadaisical about doctors' appointments and then end up in heart failure. A drug addict would use a dirty needle and then show up in the ER with a disgusting, necrotic abscess. A diabetic patient would gorge on doughnuts and white rice, then end up semiconscious from hyperglycemia. An alcoholic would binge, then turn up with seizures. Homeless patients would show up whenever it got cold out, knowing that if they said the magic words *chest pain*, they would be guaranteed a bed and hot meals for at least a day or two. Heroin addicts would come to the ER when they ran low on their supply and try to wheedle narcotics for various invented ailments.

All of these patients needed, and in some cases demanded, immediate treatment. Joanne didn't mind the medical treatment part so much, but it seemed to her that few patients took any responsibility for their role in their medical crisis. It was the sense of entitlement that drove Joanne crazy. "Patients didn't take care of themselves," she said, "and then they ended up in the ER and expected you to do everything for them."

If her son, Jeremy, had a tantrum or threw his food on the floor, as a parent she could reprimand him with a time-out, and eventually he would learn the rules. But if her patients did careless or deliberate things that ruined their health, there was no avenue for "discipline." Joanne had no choice but to take whatever her patients dished out, no matter how self-destructive.

She recalled a man who brought his kindergarten-age son to the ER. The father had given the son a firecracker to set off for a celebration. But the five-year-old couldn't coordinate throwing the lighted firecracker at the right time, and so it exploded in his hand, burning off a few fingers in the process. Joanne was overcome with anger toward this father. How could he be so stupid? What the hell had he been thinking, giving a firecracker to a five-year-old? She wanted to grab the father and shake the idiocy out of him, shake him until his bones rattled. *He* deserved to lose a few fingers, not his kid. But there was Osler's *equanimitas* again, advising doctors to curb their emotions. Joanne was required by professional duty to be neutral with him. But it made her stressful job all the more trying. It was a chore just to hold her voice steady and be civil to him.

Joanne recalled another patient, a sweet gentleman with terrible, end-stage emphysema. Every month or so, he would have an episode of difficulty breathing. His family would call 911, and the man would be intubated and brought to the ER. Eventually he would recover, and the breathing tube could be removed. Then it would happen again. The patient despised the tube in his throat and just wanted it out. He understood that the emphysema was incurable and that he would die from it. But his family bullied him into continuing treatment, and they called 911 every time, unable or unwilling to let him die.

Joanne would receive the patient in the ER each time, a tube in his trachea, and she could feel her fury toward the family members, who were letting their own issues take precedence and refusing to allow their father to die. She wanted to scream at them: *Can't you see what you are doing to your father? How can you be so goddamn selfish? This poor man wants to be at peace!* She knew, deep down, that the situation was painful for the family too, yet she was so angry that there were times when she could barely stand to make eye contact with them.

The repetitive cycles of ignorance, willful self-damage, neglect, and then entitlement, wore Joanne down. She found herself endlessly frustrated with her patients, and increasingly angry at them. She had to bite her tongue to keep from saying what she really felt. She could sense her empathy level dropping and her temper rising. The nightly glass of wine to relax became two. And then three. When she worked an overnight shift and arrived home in the brightness of the morning sun, she found that she couldn't unwind enough to sleep. And so her nightly drink also became her morning drink.

The night shifts themselves became their own torture. ER doctors, it seemed, never outgrew night work, the way internists and surgeons did as they moved along their career tracks. Seniority, per se, didn't really exist in the ER. Even the attendings who had been around for years still had to do their share of night shifts.

Even one or two nights per week could disrupt sleep patterns for the whole week, which made parenting even more difficult. Joanne realized she was facing the prospect a lifetime of lousy sleep, that she wasn't likely to have a decent night's sleep until she turned seventy. "In those days," Joanne said, "there was no support for doctors who were having a hard time. You were just expected to suck it all up."

Alcohol became her only source of relief. At first it was a way of numbing the pain at the end of a shift. Soon it became the only way to steel herself for the day to come. About five years into her post-residency career, she began to have inklings that this was a problem.

For the next two years she felt the constant presence of a little voice in the back of her head saying, *You might be an alcoholic.* She heeded it a bit, making efforts to quit. She'd white-knuckle it for a few days, but then the need for a drink would be so overpowering in the face of her stressful time in the ER that she'd go right back to her pattern.

There were no major medical mistakes that Joanne can recall, but she knows that she could have been a better doctor during those years—more patient, more empathic. She knew that she wasn't as sharp or as fast as she normally was, but she was able to get by. Still, she realized that she detested her job and that she was poisoning herself on account of it. Worse, she was putting her patients at risk.

Then one day, she arrived at work inebriated. No one noticed at first, and she grabbed a few charts and started seeing patients as usual. But within an hour, it was apparent to the nurses, doctors, interns, and orderlies all around her that she was unable to function. It was the first time she'd ever been too incapacitated to work, and now every person could see it. Stolen glances turned to whispers and then gaping stares and then finally urgent phone calls. An intervention was hastily arranged.

The chief of the emergency department was called in. "We need to draw your blood and check an alcohol level," he said firmly to Joanne. "But you have to do something about this, or you will lose your job." He said she could enroll in an outpatient rehab or a thirty-day inpatient program, but she had to do something immediately.

The best Joanne could muster was "I don't know. I'm too drunk to decide." She gathered her things with as much composure as she could rally, but it is hard to maintain a shred of dignity when you are completely plastered in front of your colleagues. The whole experience was mortifying beyond belief, a worst imaginable nightmare. But on some level, it was also a relief. She hadn't planned to quit clinical medicine entirely—the hospital ended up firing her, despite the reassurances from her boss—but this drunken episode rescued her from what had become an unending source of misery.

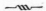

Disillusionment in medicine is a complex issue that is bandied about in attention-grabbing headlines. Just about every published survey and news article about it leads with the finding that the majority of doctors would not recommend the field to their children, or would quit if they could, or are getting MBAs in droves.[1] In fact, disillusionment is more complicated and nuanced than the media suggests. And it affects not just doctors but their patients, staff, students, and families.

Disillusionment can be a pervasive state of being, calling up complex emotions triggered by feeling that medicine wasn't what you thought it was, that your ideals of being a doctor have come into conflict with reality, and that reality is flattening those ideals to the mat. Disillusionment has many causes and components. Joanne's case illustrates what might be thought of as the purest form of disillusionment: frustration with the actual essence of taking care of patients, the feeling that many patients can't be helped or don't deserve to be helped.

Other doctors talk about external stressors that diminish the otherwise enjoyable experience of caring for patients—administrative headaches, time pressures, financial squeezes, family strains. But these all have in common the feeling of "This isn't what I bargained for when I started medical school." And they also have in common that patients feel the effects—whether subtle or major. Any doctor who is feeling anger at patients, or frustration, or boredom probably isn't doing as good a job as he could be, and may, in fact, be causing harm.

Disillusionment among doctors is nothing new. But there is a sense that it is becoming more pervasive in recent decades. To some degree, disillusionment is a built-in stage on the medical trail. There's pre-med, med school, internship, residency, clinical practice . . . and then somewhere along the line, there is disillusionment, as the rosy ideals that inspired students to enter medicine give way to the realities of daily work life.

Some of this is to be expected—for a decade or more of medical school and clinical training, the goal is to learn medicine. There is, by definition, a self-centered aspect to this, as each student has to be responsible for getting herself educated in the vast body of medical knowledge. This uphill climb is onerous, to be sure, but there is a sense of bettering yourself, with the ultimate goal of doing good for your patients.

Once the new physician is out in the working world of medicine, however, the focus necessarily has to shift outward. It is no longer about self-betterment; it's about getting the job done.

This precipitous loss of focus on personal and professional enrichment can be disorienting. Doctors, who have typically been full-time striving students for a good twenty-five years before they get their first real paycheck, often aren't prepared for the radical shift out of academic mode.

Initially, I did not notice this shift in my own career. For my first few years as a "real doctor," post-residency, I still maintained the internship mentality, that working this hard was educating me and improving my skills in an exponential manner. It took a few years to notice that the betterment curve was flattening out. Education—even though I was in an academic setting as a faculty member—was a sideline to the primary business of taking care of patients. While we did have weekly lectures and journal clubs, it was clear that this was a perk, not the sine qua non it had been for the prior decade. Doctors taking care of patients, after all, brings in revenue to the hospital; doctors sitting in a lecture—even *giving* the lecture—does not.

But finding my stride as an independently functioning physician so dominated my life in these early years that I didn't really notice this subtle but significant change. I was so busy trying to get comfortable treating the basic hypertension and diabetes of my clinic and developing my own style of practicing medicine that I didn't have time to realize that I wasn't actually learning as much as I had been.

In fact, I didn't become fully aware of it until a completely non-medical element entered my life—the cello. Shortly after my fortieth birthday, my five-year-old daughter Naava started violin lessons. I asked the violin teacher for advice on how to get a strong-willed child to practice. I expected her to discuss charts, stickers, and rewards, but instead she said, "The best way to get a child to practice is to see the parent practice."

So, taking these parental obligations concretely, I dutifully purchased a cello and signed up for my own lessons. (I thought it best not to play the same instrument but a close cousin instead.) I began to practice in the evenings as soon as my kids were tucked into bed, so that they could hear me as I conscientiously modeled my exemplary practice behavior. Not only that, I'd be a parent nonpareil, serenading my children to sleep with live classical music. No cloying baby-music CDs for us. One evening, quite early in my cellistic adventures, I was practicing at bedtime, dutifully sawing away on the four open strings—I didn't yet know how to position my fingers—when Naava called out plaintively from her bed: "Do you know any other notes?"

But the obligatory nature of practice quickly melted away, as I fell in love with the sonorous embrace of the cello. Suddenly, I was plunged back into in an avid learning environment, starting at the bottom and working my way painstakingly up the mountain. The thrill of learning and accomplishing stimulated me so much that the work was pleasurable. I found myself practicing more and more—to the detriment of keeping up with my medical journals—amazed at how much there was to learn. My desire to improve was so powerful that I practiced hungrily every single night. This pursuit of knowledge and betterment, along with an expert teacher, dedicated time and space to learn, and palpable reward for effort—reminded me of what medical school and internship had been like.

It suddenly dawned on me that this was what I was missing in my medical career now. This concentrated learning and exponential increase in knowledge was nearly absent in the real world of being a doctor. Sure, I was still learning a little here and there, but the intense gratification of getting better thanks to hard work had disappeared. In music I was clambering up over Fauré's Elegy, Bruch's *Kol Nidrei*, Schubert's Unfinished Symphony, Beethoven's first string quartet, the Bach suites—exhausted, but exhilarated. In medicine, the chronic illnesses of hypertension, diabetes, obesity, and depression remained as immutable and intractable as ever. Each "new and exciting" clinical trial was little more than a rejiggering of existing treatments with only incremental advances in the field. Nothing much seemed to change, and it all felt so dull and flavorless. But I could not articulate this loss until I rediscovered the pleasure of learning in another field.

The association became even stronger when I stumbled across an article in the *Annals of Internal Medicine* entitled "What Musicians Can Teach Doctors," which was about the intense connection between music teacher and student, the continuous one-on-one feedback.[2] It made the analogy that clinical medicine is, in some respects, a real-time performance. Doctors are onstage, in a sense, when they are with patients.

Musicians are constantly performing—whether in concert halls or in their own living rooms—always with the conscious mindset of paying attention to the performance and improving every aspect. Indeed, medical school and internship had some of that feeling, especially with senior doctors, grades, and exams to give you feedback. But all that had evaporated in the real world of medicine. There was only self-critiquing as a tool to help improve performance, and frankly, with the busyness of the hospital and the lack of a teacher waiting every week to assess my progress, it was easy to fall into a repetitive rut.

My cello teacher always warned against playing the same thing over and over just for the sake of repetition. "If you are not improving," he said, "you are getting worse." The same thing could be said about medicine.

One could certainly make the argument that this is somewhat self-centered—this desire for the stimulation of learning and betterment—but I do believe it is an under-recognized component of the disillusionment many doctors face in midcareer. And ultimately, it is patients who suffer most when their doctors are stagnating.

Whether medicine conditions us to need constant stimulation by dint of the long training or whether it simply selects for that hunger in individuals isn't clear. But after a quarter of a century of intensely learning, of having that as the basis of existence, there is an odd blandness to life without it.

—⁓—

Of course, lack of stimulation and the diminishment of the drive to improve is only one aspect of disillusionment, and one that often doesn't even register on the consciousness of many doctors. The one that does register—nearly constantly—is the aggravation of the work environment in medicine today. In a survey by the Physicians Foundation, 94 percent of nearly twelve thousand primary care doctors said that paperwork had been increasing in the previous three years. Most said that this was directly taking away from time with patients.[3]

In January of 2010, before health-care reform was signed into law, surveys indicated that a third to a half of doctors would consider closing their practices or retiring early if the bill was passed.[4] The threat—real or imagined—of additional regulations, paperwork, and administrative hassles was enough to make a lot of doctors want to throw in the towel. The specter of half the medical force dropping out, of patients wandering endlessly in search of medical care, was played out in the news with postapocalyptic melodrama worthy of Wagner.

But what people tell surveyors they will do bears only a tenuous relationship to what they actually do. The health-care reform bill passed, and there was no mass exodus of physicians. Patients did not die in the streets. Doctors—like all people—vent their frustrations to pollsters, but these sentiments don't necessarily reflect how they will behave. The polls do, however, confirm that disillusionment and frustration are nearly universal among doctors, at least to some degree. Even if doctors aren't exiting in droves, the fact that so many *think* of leaving is dire. For patients, and for society in general, this is critical to address.

There are very few studies quantifying how many doctors quit clinical medicine because of disillusionment. One of the few done indicated that general internists left medicine at a higher rate than subspecialists. Overall, about one in six general internists had left internal medicine by midcareer (for any reason), compared with one in twenty-five specialists.[5]

This would come as no surprise to internists and other primary caregivers, who feel themselves disproportionately burdened by the administrative yoke of medicine. They are referred to as the gatekeepers of medicine, but they often feel more like medicine's dumpsters. Any new clinical mandate (for instance, that every patient must be asked about seat-belt use or domestic violence or lead paint) nearly always falls on the shoulders of the primary caregivers. When patients have trouble with their insurance companies over denied claims, prior approvals, or prescription plans, they turn to their primary caregivers.

Specialists have the luxury of selecting which patient concerns they wish to handle; they can draw their practices' scope as widely or as narrowly as they desire. Whatever they don't want to deal with, they simply toss back to the primary care docs, who have to take whatever comes to them (and who, of course, get paid far less than the specialists).

For primary care doctor and specialist alike, though, the most onerous burden is paperwork. American doctors and their medical practices face an inordinate amount of paperwork by the mere fact of having to deal with multiple insurance companies, each with its own byzantine rules. A recent study showed that U.S. medical practices spend ten times as many hours on nonclinical administrative duties as comparable Canadian practices.[6]

The problem is that this paperwork eats directly into patient care, since doctors are not allotted time for this work and rarely have enough support staff to help with it. The 4.3 hours every week that each primary care doctor in a small private practice must spend haggling with insurance companies[7] is 4.3 hours not spent with patients. This doesn't even include time required for documentation (writing in charts), checking labs, ordering tests, and communicating with other members of the health-care team.

A study of hospitalists (doctors who work only with patients admitted to the hospital) showed that they spend only 17 percent of their day in direct patient care; that is, actually physically with a patient.[8] The vast majority of their time (64 percent) is spent documenting, reviewing medical records, communicating with other staff members, and handling paperwork. For physicians, this "indirect patient care" is perceived as time they are spending on patients' cases, but for patients, this indirect care is invisible. Patients are aware only of the time they actually see their doctor, and it feels like almost nothing—typically just a few minutes a day on rounds. The patients, rightly, feel shortchanged.

Doctors also feel shortchanged by this. Most would much rather be with their patients than sitting at a computer typing notes about them. But because there is so much documentation and paperwork to do, there is intense time pressure on doctors to rush their histories and physicals. All the doctors I know wish they could have more time with the patients and less time writing these hundreds and thousands of notes—though, as I was to discover, any one of these notes could become critical once lawyers start poking around.

In a commentary I once wrote about how the computer has become a wedge between doctors and patients, I described the hospital as "the 21st century equivalent of the 1950s secretarial pool: doctor after doctor hunched over the desk, dutifully pounding away at their keyboards."[9] This is an immensely disillusioning experience for people who entered medicine to help others. The paperwork and documentation requirements—which continue to increase—feel like a ball and chain keeping doctors away from their patients and from the ideals that brought them to the medical field in the first place.

—⁂—

Beyond the paperwork, medical care itself can seem like a never-ending time commitment. Medicine has always been a full-time occupation, even for part-timers. Patients do not confine their illnesses to business hours, so night and weekend work is part of the territory, especially for primary care doctors. Doctors understand that this is built into medicine, and it is part of the commitment for which they earn respect, as well as a salary higher than that of many other professions.

Nevertheless, as our society ages and illnesses become more chronic and complex (most people in developed countries no longer die of simple infections), the time required for medical care is expanding, and this spillover is affecting more and more doctors' personal lives. It can be hard for physicians to voice a complaint about this, because it is part of the professional commitment. Yet at some point, this spillover can eat away at marriages, time with children, sleep, and sanity. Even when doctors are doing the clinical medicine that they enjoy and find meaningful, when it erodes the rest of their lives, they become disillusioned. Many consider quitting.

A group of researchers followed geriatricians—primary care doctors who take care of older patients—to see how much medicine crept into their personal lives. They found that nearly eight additional hours of medical care—patient care outside of office hours—was given each week, mostly in phone calls with patients and families.[10] A similar study of internists showed that 20 percent of their total work was spent after hours.[11] This is equivalent to almost a full additional day of work every week.

It's hard to imagine a lawyer or plumber providing eight extra hours of work each week for clients just because it's the right thing to do. And of course, it is impossible to imagine lawyers or plumbers not billing—heavily!—for it. But that is the expectation of medicine. Again, for most doctors, this is an understood part of the deal, but as these extra hours increase, they have a distinct negative impact. Eight more hours of work comes directly from the rest of the doctor's life—family time, sleep, exercise, recreation. (Based on the standard American work schedule, that's ten full weeks each year.) Many doctors' lives are suffering because of this. And yet when your beeper goes off, or the hospital calls, or the answering service wakes you, there's no other option. You must attend to it.

Because of the rigors and length of their training, many doctors start families later than other professionals. The "junior" swath of physicians—those in their thirties and forties—enter their prime career-building years at the very same time they are starting families.

A generation or two ago, there *was* no work-life balance issue, since most doctors were men, and they usually had wives who were home with the children. Today, of course, nearly half of all doctors are women,[12] and almost none—men or women—have spouses handy to be home with the kids full-time. Additionally, most young male doctors recoil at the experiences of their predecessors; they don't want to miss out on their children.

The desire to have control over one's working hours—and especially those after-hours hours—is behind the trend of medical students drifting away from primary care specialties (internal medicine, family medicine, pediatrics, gynecology). Increasingly, students choose to stay—as the jargon has it—on the ROAD: radiology, ophthalmology, anesthesiology, and dermatology.[13] This trend is far more alarming than the fears raised by the health-care reform bill. Doctors here are voting with their feet and moving away decisively from primary care. A survey of more than seven thousand physicians showed the highest burnout rates in front-line fields—internal medicine, family medicine, and emergency medicine. It also noted that doctors as a group demonstrate more burnout symptoms than workers in other fields.[14] Many patients—and many doctors—are asking themselves, *Who will be my doctor when I need one?*

—⟋⟍⟍—

Disillusionment among doctors has a variety of effects. For the majority, it leads to low-level dissatisfaction and grumbling as a baseline to daily life. For some, it creates a full-blown bad temper, the type of physician both patients and fellow staff members quickly learn to avoid. There can be disruptive behavior, angry outbursts, and outright medical errors. A few doctors, of course, leave medicine and find careers elsewhere.

Some, like Joanne, turn to alcohol and drugs, a situation with substantial risk for patient harm. About 10 to 15 percent of all doctors will have issues with substance abuse at some point in their careers.[15] The causes of substance abuse are multifactorial. There may be genetic components or situations where drugs are used to enhance academic or professional performance or to stay awake. But the large majority of these doctors—like the general population—start out by using these drugs to self-medicate the painful symptoms of depression, stress, burnout, and disillusionment.

Clinical depression is a specific medical diagnosis that falls outside the discussion of this chapter, but the facets of disillusionment that lead doctors to "poison" themselves—as Joanne described it—are critically important because patients ultimately pay the price. It is one of the most powerful examples of how doctors' emotions directly affect medical care.

Because there are often few outlets for doctors to work through their disillusionment—other than staff-room gripings—quick relievers of the pain are sought. Alcohol (being legal) and prescription drugs (being easily available) are the top methods of self-medication for doctors. They rapidly take the edge off the pain. Of course, the source of the pain is continuous, so the self-medication becomes continuous and usually increases. Drug tolerance and physical addiction can quickly follow. Disillusionment also feeds on itself. When doctors feel as though they are falling short of the perfection that both they and society expect, when they feel that they are not the doctors they initially set out to be, the pain of disillusionment grows.

Of all the medical fields that face substance-abuse issues in their ranks, two stand head and shoulders above the others—anesthesiology and emergency medicine.[16] Joanne's story certainly attests to the stresses of the emergency room. Anesthesia—despite offering the cushy appeal of being on the ROAD—can be party to excessive stress. The hours and pay can be good, but the stakes are much higher than in the other ROAD careers.

An old hospital maxim is, "when the surgery goes well, you compliment the surgeon, but when the surgery goes badly, you blame the anesthesiologist." Anesthesiologists spend their days with the lives of patients literally in their hands. They are controlling the breathing and the heart rates of their anesthetized patients. When things go wrong in anesthesia, they go wrong in a catastrophic way.

Of all the medical specialties, anesthesiology has the widest access to the most addicting medications. All day long, anesthesiologists are handling heavy-duty tranquilizers, narcotics, and anesthetics. It's not hard to see how daily stress and easy access to such drugs is a dangerous combination.

Even without the complicating factor of substance abuse, stress alone can be damaging. In fact, one study found that disruptive behavior, inefficiency, and medical errors occurred just as frequently in stressed, burned-out doctors who were not substance abusers as they did in those who did have substance-abuse issues.[17]

Burnout also leads to a large swath of physicians who aren't as empathic toward their patients as they could be. These doctors don't listen as carefully or thoroughly as they should, and they may brush off patients' concerns. Like Joanne, they may be overwhelmed by anger and frustration. Such characteristics directly affect patients.

There is also a growing body of evidence to suggest that burned-out and emotionally fatigued doctors commit more medical errors.[18] Measuring this precisely is quite difficult, but the higher doctors score on measures of burnout, the more errors they admit to making. In contrast, doctors who are more engaged in their work and life report fewer errors.[19]

A seminal study by the Rand Corporation followed twenty thousand patients and their doctors for two years.[20] These were patients with ordinary chronic illnesses—diabetes, hypertension, heart disease, and depression—not acutely ill patients in the hospital. Patients and doctors alike were extensively interviewed. One of the most intriguing findings of the study was that patients were much more likely to take their prescribed medications when they were cared for by doctors who were satisfied with their jobs and lives. This is one of the first studies that directly linked doctors' inner feelings (as opposed to their concrete actions) with improved medical outcomes in patients.

—⟡—

When I think about the times I've been most stressed in my job, I realize that some of the absolute worst moments have occurred at the nexus of work life and family life. In fact, they often take place at the precise moment I am leaving the hospital to pick up my children.

One day, when I was already in my coat, bag packed, hand poised to flick off the light switch, there was the dreaded knock on the door. It was one of my patients with diabetes, worried about a small ulcer on her skin that she thought might be infected. I stood frozen in my tracks, feeling a metal vise click in place around my temples. My patient needed help—skin infections in diabetics can be life-threatening—but if I stayed with her for the time it took to do a proper evaluation, my children would be left stranded.

The vise closed steadily tighter, squeezing from both sides. Every moment I spent with my patient would directly subtract from time with my children. I could have sent her to the ER and gone on my way, but I knew that the ER would be a ten-hour ordeal for her. She'd be evaluated by doctors who didn't know her, who'd have to start from scratch to piece together her complicated medical history. They'd probably end up overordering tests to compensate. She'd probably spend the night in the ER. I knew that she had a family to tend to and that she couldn't afford extra medical bills. I couldn't bear to put her through all that.

In the end, I did what most physicians do—I tried to do both things and did neither very well. I rushed through an exam with my patient, attempting to accomplish the bare minimum of adequate medical care, and then I rushed to daycare, hoping the minutes would stretch so that I would be only a little bit late. I sprinted the whole way, arriving flustered, sweaty, angry, out of breath, still second-guessing my medical assessment of my patient's infection, arriving to see dejected children and tight-lipped, annoyed teachers who'd had to delay their return to their own families.

This feeling of being caught, of not having control over a situation, of having family life sacrificed, of being damned if you do and damned if you don't is what makes so many doctors want to quit.[21] The fundamental issue is that our medical system places doctors in impossible situations and thinks nothing of it. It is somehow a given in medicine that doctors are expected to be in two places at once or to do two different things at the same time. This basic premise accounts for much of how the system survives, without much consideration for the effects on the doctors or their patients. But it doesn't have to be this way. A simple scheduling example illustrates this.

For as long as I can remember, medical residents have had a conference at noon followed by a clinic that starts at one. Noon conference is on the seventeenth floor of the hospital building. Clinic is on the second floor of the ambulatory care building. The hallway connecting these buildings is the length of two city blocks. The elevators in each building are always crammed, especially during lunchtime. In the hospital building in particular, the doors almost always open to reveal a sardined elevator. Typically, you have to wait for five or six to go by before you could exhale all remaining breath and shoehorn yourself in, becoming more intimate with fellow hospital staff than you'd been the night before with your spouse. Alternatively, you could jog down nineteen flights of stairs. (The seventeenth floor of the hospital is actually on the nineteenth floor, because the first floor is on the third floor. Don't ask.)

Conferences are an integral part of education, so to prevent residents from skipping out of noon conference, attendance is taken and absentees disciplined. Residents have a responsibility to their patients, so if the residents arrived late to clinic, they are disciplined for tardiness. Somehow, everyone seemed to manage. The schedule had always been that way, and no one ever thought much about it

"We've basically set them up to fail," a new residency program director told me. The minute she described it that way, I saw the situation differently. Although everyone *seemed* to manage, in fact, no one was managing at all. Residents would try to sneak out of conference a few minutes early in order to get to clinic on time. Or they would tiptoe into clinic via a side door so no one would notice them coming in late. They'd cram lunch while flattened in the elevators, then sprint through the halls.

We'd created an impossible situation for them: they were required to attend a conference that finished at 1:00 in one place and also to be hard at work at 1:00 in another place that was a quarter of a mile and two elevators away from the first. Short of being beamed down *Star Trek*–style, the resident was doomed to disappoint at one end or the other.

So the program director changed clinic to begin at 1:15 for the residents. Not exactly rocket science, but no one had thought of this in the twenty years I'd been at Bellevue. Magically, everyone now seems to be punctual. (If only some of the other challenges of medicine could be solved as simply . . .)

Being set up to fail describes much of how modern medicine works (or doesn't work) and why so many doctors feel overwhelmed, frustrated, and eventually disillusioned.

—ᴍᴍ—

But then, there is someone like Herdley Paolini, a psychologist whose petite build and soft-spoken manner belie her eighteen-wheeler energy. The type of energy that would propel a nineteen-year-old who had been raised in a traditional Brazilian family where women didn't leave the home until marriage to voyage thousands of miles on her own to pursue her academic dreams. She managed to raise the funds to embark on an adventure that was beyond her financial means, convince a conservative father to come round to her point of view, successfully navigate life in the foreign United States, and excel in her field of psychology. Passion, persuasion, and creativity allowed her to buck the system, succeed in uncharted territory, and keep her serenity and good humor intact—all without alienating those she cared about. These skills presaged her ultimate, unexpected career niche.

Hospitals traditionally refer "impaired" physicians like Joanne to outside programs for help. They don't much want to step into the muck. But in 2002, Florida Hospital in Orlando decided to start a proactive wellness program. The term *wellness* has a ring of new-age hokiness to many physicians, but it's the idea that being well is more than just the absence of disease. Being well is finding yourself on the positive side of the ledger, with actual happiness and fulfillment in life in addition to physical health. It seems fairly intuitive that people who are satisfied overall in their lives will do better at their jobs than people who are miserable and disillusioned. That satisfaction can come from many aspects of life—career, family, hobbies, spirituality, exercise, having a meaningful life philosophy.

This may sound like stuff that should fall into the personal sphere of life, not the professional sphere. But the CEO of Florida Hospital had practical concerns about physician disillusionment. Good doctors were quitting, and this was destructive to morale, not to mention terrible for patients. So he created this wellness program to proactively help physicians. Unfortunately, barely any of the doctors acknowledged its existence; even fewer showed up to any of its programs.

Then one of the doctors on the organizing committee remembered the psychologist in Michigan who'd helped him through a difficult time in his life. "She's the person you need," he told the CEO.

When Florida Hospital called Herdley and offered her the job, she said no. She had been living in Michigan for seventeen years, was managing a thriving private practice, and had children in high school. But they pressed her to at least come for a visit.

When Herdley arrived, she was impressed by the CEO's commitment to this idea of wellness. She'd never seen such robust support coming directly from the top. There would be no red tape, he promised her. She would be free to create the program she wanted, and he would personally assist in removing any obstacles she encountered.

Intrigued by this unique opportunity, Herdley uprooted her family and moved to Florida. But before making a single move to create the program, Herdley decided to shadow the doctors of the hospital. For eight uninterrupted months, she ate breakfast with them; followed them on rounds; scrubbed in for surgeries; spent time in the clinics, the emergency room, the radiology suite, the doctors' lounge. She embedded herself in the doctors' world. "I learned the language they used," she said. "I saw how their experiences pinned them down."

She observed a lot of what Joanne had experienced: how the emotional complexities of patient care could wear down even the most committed doctor. There was more busywork than meaningful time with patients. There were all sorts of competing interests—from insurance companies to hospital administration to commercial pressures—that were never addressed. The demands and liabilities of medicine were squeezing out the affirmations and rewards. She saw how the medical system seemed to milk out the last bits of humanity between doctors and patients, turning them both into commodities to be tallied, measured, and codified. Doctors had no training in how to deal with this, and there were certainly no tools provided for them.

In the evenings, Herdley devoured every piece of research she could find about disillusionment and doctors' socialization. She read up on the sociology of medicine, the details of medical training, even the history of medicine. She ended up with ten massive notebooks and a conclusion that the system had done a profound disservice to doctors, and, by extension, to patients. Doctors certainly had a role in the creation of this system, but they were the ones now suffering the results and not able to give patients their best. "There was little joy left in medicine," she said. "The general population of doctors was miserable, and many of them couldn't even see it. What they needed to thrive wasn't being provided."

Her first task was to create a safe space for doctors to talk and share experiences. She set up a weekend retreat for doctors entitled Art of Medicine—Relationships. She decided to obtain CME (continuing medical education) certification for the program so that doctors could use her program for their annual licensing requirements. When she submitted her proposal to the CME office for approval, it came back with a terse reply: *What does this have to do with medicine?*

If Herdley were a trial lawyer, she would have been able to turn to the jury and say, "I rest my case." The CME office had unwittingly demonstrated precisely what the problem was.

Not only the CME office, though. *Everyone* thought she was crazy. She was told repeatedly that no one would attend such a drippy, touchy-feely sort of thing, especially something with *relationships* in the title. But Herdley's months of preparation and personal investment paid off. The doctors trusted her and believed that she had genuine concern for their welfare. They didn't view her as the usual administrative window-dressing they were accustomed to.

Thirty doctors attended the retreat, ordinary staff doctors who would never consider seeing a psychologist or joining something as sappy as a support group. But these ordinary staff doctors were bursting at the seams with stories and experiences that they wanted— *needed*—to share.

Herdley's retreat has become an established annual event at Florida Hospital. Spouses and children are invited to attend so that families can also have quality time together during the breaks. This sort of peer support continues during the year with Finding Meaning in Medicine groups, based on the work of Dr. Rachel Naomi Remen.[22] Doctors gather at one another's homes to share stories and reconnect with the parts of medicine that often get lost in the morass of practice.

In addition to these directly supportive efforts, Herdley organizes social, cultural, and education events for the physicians as well as the rest of the medical staff, designed to demonstrate the hospital's commitment to the importance of staff members' well-rounded lives. When Herdley sent out a notice proposing a staff musical concert (Physicians in Concert), her fax machine broke down under the weight of the replies. Nearly five hundred people attended the concert, which has become another annual event.

When I was invited by Herdley to address the Florida Hospital staff, the lecture was held not in the typical bland auditorium but in the local art museum. The program included dinner, a tour of the museum, autographed books for everyone, plus the CME credit needed to maintain licensure. None of these perks were "necessary" for a standard academic lecture, but they transformed the entire experience for everyone—including me.

The mere fact that the hospital was devoting resources and energy to physicians' quality of life seemed to have a salutary effect on the staff. The doctors are proud of the program and regard it as a mark of the hospital's enlightenment, not as a source of shame. There is a modest budget from the hospital, but most of the money comes from the doctors themselves, who contribute willingly.

Herdley also offers private counseling to physicians on everything from daily frustration to family issues to substance abuse to full-fledged burnout. Herdley's message to the staff is "I'm available to accompany you on your journey," whether it be in the hospital, with a patient, or in private life. Herdley also makes a point of meeting individually with every single new doctor hired. She wants to make each of them aware from the get-go of the hospital's commitment to the staff. She wants them all to know where her door is and that there is a place to turn to even for small things. Certainly before things become overwhelming.

The hallmark of the success and acceptability of her program is that 99 percent of the physicians who attend counseling do so voluntarily, based on the positive experiences of colleagues; they don't wait to be ordered into treatment by a supervisor after something terrible happens.

The program is not a panacea for all the ailments of medicine, but it is a powerful investment in the idea that physicians are whole people and that the odds of their providing superb medical care are enhanced by tending to not just their medical skills but also their emotional and psychological well-being. Many such programs are getting good results.[23]

Little of this existed when Joanne was going through her crisis. Nobody was interested in hearing from doctors who were having doubts, who were overwhelmed, who were unraveling. "Suck it up" was the modus operandi. Real doctors were supposed to be immune to this sticky side of medicine or, at the very least, able to handle it discreetly, covertly, alone.

For Joanne, her crisis was a solitary experience, a lonely buildup of misery that came to the attention of her colleagues and hospital only when her world came crashing down. And even then, the only concrete action the hospital took was to remove her from the premises and then fire her. The exact opposite of what Herdley Paolini would prescribe.

For Joanne, leaving the emergency room behind was cataclysmic and humiliating. But it was also a relief. She described it as throwing off an enormous, painful weight. Joanne realized that she was utterly miserable in her job, that what she'd loved as a resident had eroded away. The joy of solving medical mysteries and helping patients get better had been erased, replaced by a bitter and festering resentment of patients who didn't seem to care about their health and simply tossed their problems into her lap.

On March 5, 1993—twenty-four hours after she'd been escorted out of the emergency room inebriated—Joanne checked herself into a thirty-day rehab. She flung herself at recovery with the same energy she'd applied to her medical studies. She discovered that her inner energy and reserve were still there, despite the recent difficult years. And, as in her academic sphere, her determination and hard work paid off: the rehab was successful on the first go-round. In the two decades since the intervention at the hospital, she has not had another drink.

During her rehabilitation, Joanne had to wrestle with who she was. Like all of her family, she'd always—and only—defined herself as a doctor. Now what exactly was she? Was she an ex-doctor? A failed doctor? A non-doctor?

Contrary to what she might have expected, she actually did not feel like a failure as a doctor. She could look back at her years in medicine—short of the last few abysmal weeks—and feel satisfied that she had delivered competent medical care to her patients. But she also had to accept the fact that she was completely burned out from clinical medicine, disillusioned with the realities of trying to help the challenging patients for whom the ER was a primary source of medical care.

It was during this recovery time that Joanne began to appreciate the irony of her situation. She had been so intensely angry at her patients for their self-destructive behavior, and yet she'd done the exact same thing. This perspective gave her more sympathy for those patients and brought her some peace about her decision to leave clinical medicine.

Though her health was returning, she still found herself afloat in terms of career. She knew she could not be the kind of doctor who worked directly with patients. But with support from her family, and with her own research, she learned of the myriad other ways that doctors could use their medical knowledge productively. Joanne enrolled in a master's program in public health and found that she loved it. The idea of improving the health of large populations by addressing such broader issues as immunization, screening, access to care, and patient education was appealing. This was how she could help patients *avoid* ending up in the ER. It was the best medical education experience she'd ever had. She was able to engage in improving people's health without the interfering black shadows of frustration and anger.

There weren't any jobs in public health available when she graduated, so she started doing medical writing to support herself and Jeremy. She found that she was good at it and could address the medical issues that she felt were important. She ended up getting a job in the field of continuing medical education. It wasn't what she had planned, but it has turned out to be a gratifying way to put her medical and public health experience to good use—helping other doctors stay current in the medical field. This was her way to be a real doctor:

she was able to help patients by helping their doctors, and she didn't have to deal with the brutal frustrations of the ER.

Most doctors who are burned out, though, do not shift careers. They stay in medicine because it is the only thing they know. For those lucky enough to find someone like Herdley Paolini, they often find a workable way of continuing. Peer support from colleagues or working with a psychologist or psychiatrist can help a doctor reconnect with what was important in medicine in the first place. Other doctors need to make changes in their work lives—switch practice settings, cut back on hours—or in their personal lives. Focusing more on family, scraping together a little time for clarinet or basketball, or finally attacking *Ulysses* can strengthen the girders for them to face the challenges at work.

It also takes creativity, flexibility, and commitment on the administrative side to modify some of the structural frustrations of medicine. Simple things—like shifting the clinic start time from 1:00 to 1:15—can go a long way. Bigger things—like on-site child care with flexible hours—can be lifesaving. But it remains a sad reality that many doctors will simply live with the festering burn of dissatisfaction, a burn that will ultimately be felt by their patients.

Joanne considers herself lucky to have found a compromise that allows her to help patients and doesn't eat away at her soul. Plus, there are other perks. "I get to go to sleep every single night," she said. This may seem as mundane as breathing for most people, but for doctors, nurses, and other caregivers who have worked the night shift, the simple act of sleeping each and every night is a victory akin to reaching the Promised Land after forty years in the desert. "And," she told me with a grateful sigh, "no one has thrown up on me in years."

Julia, part six

On a warm October morning, as I sat in my clinic office sorting through reams of lab results, the telephone rang. It was the cardiologist from Columbia University's transplant program.

"I thought you'd want to know," he said, "that Julia got a heart last night."

Even today, I find myself at a loss for words to describe the flood of emotions that overcame me at that moment. Eight years of suppressed fear and anxiety unshackled with a force of tearing metal, and a visceral cry of elation erupted. I burst out of my office and tore down the hall of the clinic, hollering, "She got a heart! Julia got a heart!"

I collared every colleague, intern, student, patient, orderly, and administrator I stumbled across. I danced up and down the halls, announcing the news to every sentient being within a hundred yards. The joy was all-encompassing, and my desire to share had a surging force of its own.

I realized that the network of people invested in Julia's case had blossomed steadily over the years. All of my close friends knew about Julia from all the times I'd confided in them about her tragic predicament. I had to call each of them to tell them the exciting news.

And then there were my writing buddies and editors who knew Julia from my books and articles. I had to contact all of them. The reporters who had written about Julia for newspapers and magazines—I had to let them know. And then of course I had to call my parents and my husband, who had all been following Julia's progress over the years. (I would even celebrate with my children later on that evening. They'd watch, slightly baffled, as their no-sugar-before-bedtime mother dished out gargantuan scoops of ice cream, plus sprinkles—chocolate *and* multicolored—while regaling them with the immunological science behind organ transplantation.)

It seemed like the world was celebrating, and, damn it, why not? Julia deserved it. For all that she suffered—with dignity, grace, and heartbreak—she deserved the biggest party we could throw. This unassuming woman from rural Guatemala now had people cheering her on from Boston to Israel to California to Canada to Florida to England.

When I finally sat back down in office to catch my breath, I realized that there were tears streaming down my cheeks. I was so overcome with joy that I hadn't even realized I was crying. Those tears that I'd held back for so long—they were finally here.

Tears of joy might rank as one of the most sublime experiences in the human emotional spectrum. It's rare to feel so rapturously happy that one is completely overcome. Certainly it's a rare commodity in medicine. So rare that it hardly merits mention. But here it was—honest-to-goodness joy.

As the headiness of the morning gradually began to settle, I contemplated the rarity of joy in our profession. In the months that I attend on the wards, I watch the interns and residents enmeshed in caring for patients, ricocheting from frustration to fear to anger. There are certainly moments of pride, pleasure, even fun. But pure joy almost never comes up.

The only time I ever hear *joy* and *hospital* in the same breath is in the poem that I read aloud frequently to my students, John Stone's "Gaudeamus Igitur" (Latin for "Therefore, let us rejoice"). And this is the poem that came to my mind the morning of Julia's new heart.

> . . . and you will walk triumphantly
> in purest joy
> along the halls of the hospital
> and say Yes to all the dark corners
> where no one is listening.[1]

But now people were listening. After eight frightening years with Julia's life on the line, people had finally listened. The world had finally listened. It had opened its heart and given her a second chance at life. I was proud to bursting of Bellevue Hospital and the scores of dedicated staff who'd slogged through overwhelming bureaucracy and resistance to make this transplant happen. It was a miracle against all human odds. I was grateful to the family of the twenty-two-year-old bicyclist killed by a taxi, who in their grief had the generosity of spirit to donate his heart. I felt indebted to Julia's parents and especially her sister Claribel, who had imbued her with the dogged survival instinct that brought her to this day. I was ecstatic for Julia's two children, who would not have to negotiate life motherless.

Julia finally had a heart.

Gaudeamus igitur!

CHAPTER 7

Under the Microscope

Every intern and resident has a hierarchy of the worst pages to receive. For me, when I was a resident, the most dreaded number to see on my beeper was 3015, because being paged by the ER always meant a new admission and more work. Extension 4878 was probably next on my list, because anything to do with the prison ward meant hauling myself up to the nineteenth floor and going through the four sets of metal gates and a security check. Even the smallest task would entail a thirty-minute ordeal.

But 5031 was a number I didn't recognize. When I called back, my hierarchy of worst pages was hastily re-ordered. Risk Management. The department that no doctor ever, ever wants to hear from.

As a resident, I was still fresh enough in the medical field that I didn't have much of an idea of what Risk Management was. The term itself had a queasy, corporate-speak veneer that felt entirely out of place in our world where most things possessed organic, no-nonsense titles, like *admitting office, operating room, medical records, hematology lab,* and *coffee shop.* All most residents knew was that Risk Management equaled lawyers. It was located in that inner sanctum of the hospital where the suits dwelled, where the atmosphere was whisper-quiet, where the walls were paneled with wood, and not a soul possessed urine samples in their pockets, bags under their eyes, or pus on their shoes.

When I dialed 5031, a crisp administrative voice informed me that my presence was requested for a chart review. I glanced around

173

the intensive care unit where I was working that month. There were twelve patients on ventilators, some in septic shock, some in heart failure, some infected with more pathogens than I had fingers, some having just coded, some just shy of coding. My first response was an equally crisp "I'm a trifle busy at this moment. You see, there is the small matter of these critically ill patients here in the ICU." I was nearing the end of residency, the peak of my self-assuredness, and I had a well-honed impatience for any administrator type whose feet had never been dirtied in the clinical trenches.

"Fine," the voice replied. "We shall send the lawyer to the ICU."

Lawyer?

If there is a sucker-punch for a doctor, the word *lawyer* is it. I dashed to the nearest sink and started washing my face and hands, trying to scrub away the overnight grubbiness. My white coat was grimy, my scrubs had been slept in, my hair was practically in dread-locks. I grabbed toothpaste from the patient supply cart and hurriedly rinsed my mouth out. I buttoned my grimy white coat and hoped for the best.

The lawyer arrived promptly. She wore a trim herringbone suit, stylish heels, and a shimmering white blouse that was so pristinely immaculate that I found myself staring at it, somewhat dumbly, until she gently cleared her throat.

She turned out to be quite pleasant—I guess I'd been expecting more of a linebacker type. She apologized for taking up my time, but there was a family who was considering a lawsuit. "Nothing's been filed yet," she told me, "and it may very well come to nothing. Nevertheless, the hospital feels it is prudent to be prepared."

Prudent. Not a word that offered much comfort.

"Therefore, we are reviewing the chart with all personnel involved in the case."

"All?" I asked, looking at the voluminous chart in her hand.

"Yes. Every one." She smiled charitably at me, the way a preschool teacher might smile at a toddler who still doesn't know the words to the cleanup song. "And we need to read over every last word in this chart." She set it down on the table, where it landed with an ominously muffled thud. We were sitting in a conference room off the ICU. The table was Formica, sticky from a month of Chinese take-out and round-the-clock coffee. Surplus packets of low-sodium soy sauce and Sweet'N Low—some packets used, others with life still in them—formed an ignoble mound at the far end. The lawyer remained tactfully focused on the business at hand.

She opened the chart. "Our job is to go through every single page of this chart. You will point out your notes. We will go through your notes, word by word, making sure everything is clear. Sound okay?"

No, it did not sound okay. A quick shot of soy sauce and Sweet'N Low sounded a hell of a lot more okay than parsing through my writing with a lawyer.

"We're on your side," she reminded me, which did surprisingly little to calm my agitation.

We got right down to business, since the very first page of the chart was in my handwriting—Resident Admitting Note. It was a case of a twenty-three-year-old woman—Mercedes—who had come to the hospital with a simple headache. She was friendly and engaging and the picture of health, with thick brown hair that surrounded her glowing complexion. We liked each other immediately, not least because we were only a few years apart in age. The case took on early notoriety, because her condition rapidly and inexplicably deteriorated and then I diagnosed her with Lyme disease, something exceedingly rare for a person who hadn't set foot out of the inner city. I became something of a local hero in the hospital for even considering such an unexpected disease, much less diagnosing it. Her treatment was altered to a Lyme disease protocol, and she promptly recovered. Her case was triumphantly presented at a departmental meeting, and I invited her to attend, even though she'd been discharged and was already back running after her two little children.

Patients weren't usually part of such conferences. I suppose I wanted palpable evidence of my accomplishment, but it was also that I wanted her to be part of this victory lap. It was her victory, really. That Friday-afternoon conference felt like a celebration.

On Monday—not even seventy-two hours after our conference— Mercedes awoke with another headache, so she returned to the ER and was sent to radiology for a CT scan. Midway through the scan, she suddenly went into cardiac arrest. The code team crammed into the CT suite to revive her, but her pupils were already fixed and dilated. Her brain had begun to herniate down through the base of her skull due to severe inflammation.

By the time Mercedes was wheeled up to the ICU, she was brain-dead. I wasn't on call that evening, so normally I wouldn't have known about the cataclysmic turn of events till the next morning on rounds. But the condition of one of my other patients had been gnawing at me, and so I telephoned the ICU from home—something I rarely did—to see if his vent settings could be optimized. That's when I learned that Mercedes, whom I'd seen robust and healthy on Friday, was now dying.

It was impossible to sleep once I'd heard. A restlessness seized hold of me, twisting my insides, grinding my thoughts. Finally I pulled on some clothes and walked over to the hospital in the prickling darkness, needing to see with my own eyes. It was a devastating sight—Mercedes, looking for all the world like a healthy twenty-three-year-old woman, hooked up to a ventilator while the overhead monitors charted the relentless swelling of her brain. She was surrounded by her extended family. The Catholic chaplain—a balding, rotund man in black robes—was there to administer last rites.

I remember that I opened my mouth to speak to the family. I felt that I needed to say something; I'd been the one, after all, who'd given them the confident Lyme disease diagnosis so recently. I tried to explain, to apologize, to comfort, anything. . . . But nothing came out. I simply broke down weeping, crumpling into the arms of a priest whose name I didn't even know.

The Lyme disease diagnosis collapsed beneath repeated tests that were now negative. Every test for every other disease we could think of came back negative. Every brilliant mind we could find was brought to Mercedes's bedside, but all were stumped. Even the autopsy was inconclusive. It was probably some sort of encephalitis, but the exact nature eluded our medical science.

The case was devastating to everyone involved. It took months for me to recover, and I couldn't even begin to imagine the pain and grief her family had to endure. This was a tragedy in every sense of the word, but it wasn't clear that anything had been done wrong, medically. The case was reviewed exhaustively by the medical staff and no obvious errors were found, other than that our first diagnosis was incorrect due to a false-positive result on the Lyme test and we were never able to figure out what she actually had.

Nevertheless, here I sat with a lawyer, examining every step I'd taken in Mercedes's case. The lawyer instructed me to read every word aloud to her, pausing at each acronym so that I could elaborate: "'No PMH of CVA, MI, CA, HTN, DM'—no past medical history of stroke, heart attack, cancer, hypertension, diabetes.'"

It was an excellent note by medical standards—I'd taken extra care that day to write an especially detailed note—but it suddenly looked paltry under scrutiny. Every line taken by itself seemed scrawny and pathetic. I choked over each word, digressing frequently to elaborate and explain.

"Just read what is written" came the commandment after each of my detours. Chastened, I would return to my recitation, sucking in my cheeks, which were growing more scarlet by the moment.

"At least your note is legible," the lawyer said drily as we turned the pages and arrived at the neurosurgeon's chicken scrawl. "When it's messy, the opposing lawyers can claim it says anything they want." Inwardly, I blessed Mrs. Pederson, my third-grade teacher; her falsetto during the daily singing of "The Star-Spangled Banner" used to scare the daylights out of me, but her ruler-rigid insistence on proper penmanship might wind up saving my pants in a lawsuit.

My session with the lawyer lasted almost an hour. She didn't find anything especially wrong with my notes, but she didn't seem to find anything especially right. No compliment for my clinical reasoning or my diagnostic logic. No kudos for the exceptionally thorough review of systems or the extensive neurological-exam maneuvers I'd added to the physical after combing through my neurology textbook late into the night when Mercedes was admitted.

The lawyer closed the chart, thanked me crisply, then left the room. *Did I pass?* I wanted to call out. *Did I fail? Do I have to retake the test?* But she had already rounded the corner, the heels of her corporate pumps clicking briskly along the distant hallway.

I felt like I'd been stripped naked and interrogated in front of the Inquisition, then dismissed with nothing more than a vague, noncommittal wave-of-the-hand. It was the eeriest feeling—embarrassing, inconclusive, foreboding. After that, a certain wariness seeped over me. Each time I wrote a note in the chart, I wondered how it would look to a cold, legal eye. I hesitated before each medication order, wondering not just if it was the correct thing for the patient, but whether it would look right under scrutiny. I could appreciate that extra caution might be a beneficial thing for doctor and patient alike, but there was a tinge of sleaziness to the whole process, like a third party had slithered into our space.

More than a year passed before I learned that the case had not pressed forward. No one ever told me how it was resolved, who spoke with the family, what the final assessment was. After all, I was a nobody. Just one of a flock of residents who had notes in Mercedes's chart. But I felt shaken to the core, and that unease never fully dissipated. Looking back at the situation now, I wonder about the effects of lawsuit threats on residents who are so early in their career in medicine. Nearly a quarter of all lawsuits name interns and residents among the defendants.[1] I wonder about a not insignificant swath of doctors-in-training who complete their education with an uneasiness slinking along beside them. To date, no one has studied how this affects their development as doctors, but there is certainly an increasing awareness that lawsuits are a very real part of medical training.[2]

—⟋⟍—

The next time 5031 appeared on my beeper, I was already an attending, with years more experience under my belt. When I was told the name of the patient—Yvonne Manning—I knew instantly what the issue was.

Yvonne Manning was one of the sweetest human beings to ever walk the face of this earth. She and I had the type of close doctor-patient relationship that prevailing wisdom—and hordes of well-meaning articles—assure is the best protection against lawsuits. I knew with absolute conviction that she would never file a lawsuit against me. Nevertheless, before the Risk Management lawyer even opened his mouth, I knew exactly what the case was about.

Ms. Manning was a Trinidadian woman in her mid-sixties with robust good health. I was her internist, but because she had no real medical problems, her visits offered us time to connect on many levels. We were able to discuss nutrition and exercise—things that are usually luxuries during a standard medical visit—as well as her career, her family, the latest medical breakthroughs. Though she'd never had much opportunity for formal education, she possessed an incisive intellect, hidden in part by an unassuming exterior. She'd come from a family of simple means, but with hard work and her innate skills, she managed to move herself up to a middle-management job in a personnel department. She ensured that her daughters had a middle-class life and an expectation of graduating college—which both did.

I enjoyed Ms. Manning's intelligent observations and her radiating warmth. She was someone I'd easily be friends with if we met outside the hospital, and I could tell that the feeling was mutual. Then, suddenly, breast cancer plowed into the picture. We had to turn on a dime from flu shots and cholesterol checks to chemotherapy and surgery. But because we already had a good relationship, things went as smoothly as cancer treatment allows. She and I kept in constant touch throughout every step of the three-year process, and it felt like a true partnership.

In some ways, it was one of my most gratifying experiences as a physician. I wished she didn't have this disease, of course, but her way of being and communicating allowed me to be the best doctor I could be. I was able to stand with her during this journey and help her navigate the maze of treatment, as an internist is supposed to do—something that is so often stymied for myriad reasons. The simple truth was that I adored Yvonne Manning and would have done anything for her.

I spent hours on the phone with her insurance company arguing about MRIs and pre-approvals. I convinced the social worker to approve an ambulette for her when radiation treatments made taking the bus too uncomfortable. I brought her the newspaper and her favorite lemongrass tea when she was admitted for chemotherapy. It's not that I didn't do these things for my other patients, but somehow Ms. Manning made it especially easy.

Once, she came to my office unannounced because of a vague discomfort at the site of her reconstruction. I dropped whatever it was I was doing to examine her. The incision site was slightly red and tender, though not remarkably so. It could have just been irritation, but there was a chance that it could be a post-op infection.

I paged the plastic surgeon but got only the intern, who knew nothing at all. The oncology surgeons were in the OR. The general surgeons were backed up in the ER. I knew that I had other patients waiting, but I couldn't leave this issue unresolved; Ms. Manning's only other option would have been to go to the ER and wait, and this would be very low priority in the triage system.

Then one of the clerks mentioned that the plastic surgery attending was precepting in the pediatrics clinic for the afternoon. I grabbed Ms. Manning by the arm and we took the back stairwell, then speed-walked to pediatrics. I was determined not to lose the surgeon.

We tracked him down, and in the end, it turned out to be an infection, a mild one. But we were able to catch it early, before it spread. Ms. Manning went home with antibiotic pills and warm compresses instead of getting admitted to the hospital for IV antibiotics. We hugged each other with delight over our small victory for the day—Ms. Manning for being attuned enough to notice even a slight change, and me for doggedly tracking down the surgeon. We were a team!

The cancer, unfortunately, was not curable. Despite initially responding to treatment, it kept returning and metastasizing. I helped Ms. Manning sort through her thoughts about advance directives and kept copious notes of our discussions. Her last admission ended up being at another hospital because that was where the ambulance brought her, and she wasn't very coherent by that point. But I was able to fax my detailed notes to the physician there, and he was grateful that I had so much documentation about her stated wishes.

Yvonne Manning died peacefully, without any of the aggressive interventions that she'd feared. Although I couldn't be with her in the final moments, I felt that I'd been there in spirit, helping ensure that her directives were carried out. I was so sad when she died, but also relieved that the work we'd done together had paid off. She'd been spared unnecessary suffering and died in the most comfortable circumstances possible.

Ms. Manning had two grown daughters. One was moderately involved in her care; the other only sporadically. I have a crystal-clear recollection of the day that Ms. Manning and I had discussed advance directives. We were on the oncology ward, and the clinical situation was looking grim. We'd talked for more than an hour about the limits of chemotherapy, and Ms. Manning had decided to decline further treatment and sign a DNR (do-not-resuscitate) order.

Just at that moment, the second daughter arrived. Slender, tall, stylishly dressed, she carried a bulging shopping bag from an upscale natural-foods store. I explained what her mother and I had been talking about. With precise movements, she pulled out containers of kombu seaweed soup, kukicha twig tea, macrobiotic salad, and celery juice, piling them on her mother's bedside stand. Then she spoke, tight and methodical. "I think my mother's treatment decisions are between her and her family. If you'll excuse us, Doctor."

I could see that this was my cue to exit. But I did not want to leave Ms. Manning stranded, given all that she had just confided in me. "Absolutely," I replied, getting to my feet. "My goal is to carry out your mother's wishes, especially if there comes a time when she might not be able to articulate them. Whatever she tells me now, I will write down in her chart. That way, we can be sure that we are doing what she wants."

I paused here, then felt the need to elaborate. "Not what I might want, or what her family might want, or what the insurance company might want. What *she* wants." I gave Ms. Manning a hug good-bye. The daughter pursed her lips and pointedly did not look at me as I left the room.

When the lawyer at Risk Management told me that there was a potential lawsuit from the family of Yvonne Manning about "substandard medical care," I knew that it was the daughter filing the suit. I couldn't deny that it stung, given that Yvonne Manning was one of the patients closest to my heart, for whom I'd gone the extra mile countless times. But I knew that it wasn't Yvonne doing this.

As I walked down to the Risk Management office, I recalled all the warm moments Ms. Manning and I had shared. She'd always been so appreciative of even the littlest things—the can of ginger ale, the extra box of tissues. Even at her sickest, she always took the time to thank the nurses, the therapists, the housekeepers. I also remember how relieved she was when I told her that continued treatment was optional, that she was allowed to say no. Her responses were so genuine that I knew that we had done the right thing for her, that she had received excellent and wise medical care. In my mind I whispered to her, *I know this lawsuit has nothing to do with you. It won't change my special memories of you.*

Yvonne Manning's case was one step farther in the legal process than my first brush with malpractice regarding Mercedes. Now I would be giving a deposition in the presence of the family's lawyer and the hospital's lawyer, with a court reporter transcribing every word. The fact that this took place in a hospital conference room and not a courtroom did little to assuage my discomfort.

The scene had an eerie familiarity, though now it was two lawyers—not just one—paging through a voluminous chart, asking minute questions on sentences I'd written years ago, sometimes in haste, sometimes caffeine-deprived, sometimes while juggling twenty things for ten different patients. Luckily, this was a patient I remembered vividly. There were certainly hundreds of patients that I'd never be able to summon up in my memory.

The lawyer for the Manning family pointed to my DNR note. "Did you tell the patient that she had only three to six months to live?"

"Well," I replied, in the steadiest voice I could muster, "prognosis is impossible to specify precisely. What I always say is that our information is based on averages of patients with your condition, but that this doesn't give a hard and fast number for any individual person. For some patients, the disease might progress more slowly; for others—"

"Doctor, please answer my question," the lawyer interjected. "Did you tell Yvonne Manning that she had three to six months to live?"

"When someone has recurrent metastatic cancer involving the central nervous system and is profoundly weakened from the cancer, three to six months is a reasonable starting point to begin a discussion because of the—"

"Doctor, please just answer the question."

"Well, yes. I did talk about three to six months as a rough population estimate for patients in her situation, but I am careful to emphasize that it is nearly impossible to predict individual—"

"Dr. Ofri, can you kindly provide a yes-or-no answer." This was now the hospital lawyer speaking, but he seemed equally annoyed with me.

I looked at him incredulously. Wasn't he supposed to be on *my* side? "Prognosis is not a yes/no matter," I said to him. "It's very nuanced, both on how it is estimated and how it is explained to a patient."

"This is not a medical lecture, Doctor." I've long since forgotten which lawyer snapped that retort, but the distinction was irrelevant. It was clear that both lawyers just wanted me to reply in one-word answers. Neither seemed interested in the medical care I actually gave to Ms. Manning.

I was asked by one of the lawyers to describe the day that I "mediated" between the oncologist and the patient regarding continuing treatment. I could recall that day with clarity. We were in Ms. Manning's room on 7-East. The east wing of the hospital was always bathed in crystalline morning light. It illuminated Ms. Manning from the window, and she appeared almost glowing, despite the weight loss that had carved away at her cheeks.

The oncology fellow was an Indian woman, and I remember that she wore a vermilion-colored scarf around her neck that trailed down the back of her white coat. The topic of conversation was so important that she'd brought along the other oncology fellow who knew Yvonne Manning from clinic. I was there, too, as her internist. I remember how Ms. Manning had made the situation more warm and intimate, inviting the fellows to sit on her bed. I'd pulled a chair up close. We were four women in a tight circle, almost like a small family. The oncology fellow was earnest and concerned, laying out every treatment option with all the possible risks and benefits. After each one, Ms. Manning would turn to me, and I would restate all that had just been said so that she could rethink it.

The situation was bleak. Cancer had spread to her brain for the second time, and the fellow was offering palliative chemotherapy. It wouldn't cure the disease, but it might shrink the tumors and decrease some of Ms. Manning's incapacitating headaches. But the fact that her body was already so weakened from the cancer tilted the risk-benefit ratio significantly.

After the discussion, I remember thinking that this was how medical care was supposed to be done. The patient and her doctors were a team, all involved in the discussion. We spent more than an hour talking. No one was rushed. Every question was answered. Options were offered. Realistic assessments were given. There were no platitudes, and there was compassion all around—the doctors for the patient, and the patient for her doctors. Ms. Manning understood that this couldn't be easy for the doctors, and her empathy toward us was a humanitarian gesture I'll never forget.

"The oncologists told Ms. Manning that if she didn't accept treatment she would die. Is that correct?" It was the Manning lawyer talking to me.

It took me a moment to get back to the present. "No," I said softly. "No, it wasn't that way at all. The oncologists told her that the treatment was palliative, that there might be a possibility of extending her life by a few weeks. But they didn't sugarcoat the reality. They were very gentle, but they were honest about—"

"Doctor, please answer the question."

"I *am* answering the question, but it's not a simple answer. Yes, she would die without treatment, but that was—"

"But according to the family, you recommended that she decline treatment, even though the oncologists recommended it. You encouraged the patient to refuse the treatment suggested by the specialists."

"No," I said, starting to feel confused. "That's not the way it happened. We all discussed it together. Both oncologists and I, we all talked together with Yvonne. It wasn't like they were trying to convince her of one thing, and I was trying to talk her out of it. It was a very involved discussion, and we—"

My lawyer turned to the court reporter and said, "Can we turn off the tape for a moment." Then he faced me. His voice was not unkind, but it was businesslike, and it had the overtones of a speech that he'd clearly made many times before. "Dr. Ofri, this is not a forum for you to explain your philosophy of medical care. This is a deposition and you need to answer the questions exactly as they are asked. Please do not elaborate or go on tangents. Just answer the questions."

Two weeks later, a certified package arrived at my home, containing an inch-thick stack of transcripts from the deposition. *Please review this carefully,* the note from Risk Management said. *If there are any errors in the transcription of your testimony, please mark in red and alert our office.* I kicked the package under the bed and never looked at it again.

—⁙—

Being judged stirs up a powerful and distinctive blend of emotions that can unsettle even the most stable, confident doctor. What stands out most from my two encounters with lawyers is the shivering feeling of being exposed under the bright lights of scrutiny, the sense of being naked while the examiners were clothed and comfortable.

I've tried to piece together the origins of this strong reaction. There are certainly other situations in which I've been judged that don't bother me nearly as much. Getting a letter from the IRS judging me on my tax errors and how much additional money I owe annoys me, but I don't feel exposed. Being judged every week by my cello teacher, who never minces words, actually encourages me, even if it is uncomfortable in the moment. I have a sense that he wants to help me become better, and so the judgments encourage me to redouble my efforts.

But having my medical care parsed and scrutinized by these lawyers—even the ones who were there to defend me—was an incomparably awful feeling. With Yvonne Manning's case, in particular, I felt punctured. I had invested so much of myself in her care. Despite the horrible disease, despite the inevitability of her death, I felt that she and I had worked together in a true doctor-patient partnership. I felt as though I'd come close to achieving my fullest as a physician. But this legal process seemed designed to quash that. Under the needling questions of the lawyers hovered the unspoken subtext that I was guilty of something nefarious, and the goal of the cross-examination was to trip me up and reveal it. I felt like the enemy. Even with lawyer who was on my side.

Neither Yvonne Manning's nor Mercedes's case went to trial. The lawyers negotiated among themselves, or with whomever it is that lawyers negotiate, and the charges were dropped. Unfortunately, emotions cannot be "dropped" with similar briskness. Decades later, I still retain the sting of those examinations, blunted somewhat, but there.

My experience with lawsuits seems typical. Even when malpractice suits do not move forward (and most don't), the emotional toll is taken. Sadly, this is not an insignificant issue—the majority of doctors will face some type of lawsuit during their lifetimes. The American Medical Association reports that by midcareer (defined as age fifty-five) more than 60 percent of all doctors have been involved in lawsuits.[3] This varies by specialty, with neurosurgeons and cardiac surgeons facing the most claims (nearly 20 percent face a claim each year), and pediatricians and psychiatrists the fewest (2 to 3 percent each year).[4]

One of the worst aspects of a full-blown lawsuit is its protracted nature. The process can last years, dragging out all the difficult emotions in excruciating slow motion. Two psychiatrists writing about their experience with a lawsuit described it as "a 6-year-long toothache, characterized by a baseline of constant, low-grade, gnawing discomfort punctuated by acute paroxysms of lancinating pain." They described the shadow that was cast over them for those six years. "We worked and lived in the penumbral darkness that this suit created in our lives. . . . It afforded plenty of time for smoldering doubt and meticulous, often, painful scrutiny of ourselves and of our treatment of our patient, now plaintiff."[5]

The emotional toll of being judged in this way can be overwhelming. Dealing with a lawsuit is often likened to having a death in the family. Doctors end up (often unconsciously) grieving for the doctors they used to be—the idealistic doctors who were sure that dedication, knowledge, and compassion were all that was needed, that these factors would protect them from lawsuits. But this belief is shattered, and many doctors feel embittered, having lost the joy of medicine. Many refrain from taking on patients who are perceived as challenging or who have complicated medical issues.

The striking finding is that these emotional reactions are quite consistent among doctors—whether or not a case proceeds to trial, even whether or not they are found guilty. Having a case dismissed for insufficient grounds, even being exonerated in a public court of law, does almost nothing to blunt the emotional reactions.[6] Physicians are almost always told—usually by lawyers—not to take lawsuits personally, but that is simply impossible. Nearly every doctor feels both her competence and her identity as a doctor challenged, even if the suit is entirely frivolous. The sense of being judged on the essence of who you are can override the facts of a given case.

—∿∿—

Sara Charles was a young psychiatrist, only seven years out of training. She took on a wide range of patients in her practice—from mild depressives to full-blown schizophrenics. Some of the most challenging patients were those with borderline personality disorders. Borderline patients are known for their emotional volatility and chaotic lives. Angry outbursts and unstable relationships are hallmarks, and these patients are among the most difficult to treat in psychiatric practice.

Natalie was a graduate student with borderline personality disorder who started therapy with Sara. They met regularly, working through both crises and day-to-day travails. That Natalie was keeping up with her studies and that her personal life was relatively calm were signs that things were reasonably under control. On a chilly Saturday in mid-November, two years into her ongoing therapy, Natalie climbed out her window onto the fire escape. She ascended the ladder to the roof of her building and then leaped off.

Sara was devastated when she heard the news, but also completely shocked. She had just spoken to Natalie the day before. Natalie had talked about going home to visit her family. She'd made an appointment to see Sara on Monday. These were all signs of stability, not suicidality. There had been real progress in the past few months. How could this have happened?

The fall was not fatal, but the injuries sustained were grave indeed. In the hospital, Natalie requested that her psychiatrist come see her. Sara rushed to the hospital and found a young, beautiful woman crushed. A breathing tube in her throat, body immobilized in metal contraptions, eyes jittering in fear, voice struggling to emerge, Natalie resembled—in Sara's words—"a small bird trapped cruelly in a net of steel." It was an image Sara would never forget.

Rehabilitation lasted month after painful month, and it became clear that Natalie would never walk again. Sara continued to work with Natalie during these months, helping her adjust to life as a paraplegic. Natalie was filled with both rage and guilt about her new life circumstances, and the therapy sessions were intense. In the spring, Natalie was finally discharged, and she returned to her studies. She continued in weekly therapy with Sara through the spring, then decided she wanted a new psychiatrist.

It was in October, as the autumn leaves were bathing the streets in a palette of gold and russet, that a letter from a U.S. marshal arrived on Sara's desk. The letter stated that Sara—referred to here as "the defendant"—had been negligent in Natalie's care by "not taking the Plaintiff's depression and suicidal tendencies seriously, joking about them, insulting and degrading [her] . . . which only caused the Plaintiff to go into a deeper depression . . . and ultimately to attempt to commit suicide."[7]

Joking? Degrading?

Sara had been so devastated by Natalie's case that she decided, on her own, to critically evaluate her own work as a psychiatrist. She had invested a full year of effort with a senior clinician, intensively reviewing every single session she'd had with Natalie to ensure that she hadn't missed anything. Swaths of time and thought, not to mention heart, were dedicated to Natalie's case—both then and now.

Negligent? Insulting?

It seemed to take hours for Sara to catch her breath after she got the letter. But that was nothing compared to the weeks, months, and then years of pain, self-doubt, and isolation that ensued. It seemed as though a fence of invisible mesh had walled her off from the rest of the medical world to suffer this alone.

The legal system, far from offering the relief of reasoned, factual analysis, was more akin to salt abrading a wound. The preparation for the trial was endless and inordinately taxing. Sara's medical practice, not to mention her personal life, was casually bulldozed by last-minute meetings, rescheduled depositions, urgent phone calls, and then unending waits. When the trial date finally approached, Sara steeled herself for the courtroom, working up the courage to face the oncoming assault, but then the judge went on vacation, so the trial was postponed.

Another round of preparations, of rearranged patient schedules, of bracing for the trial, and then one of the lawyers' wedding came up, and the whole thing was kicked down the road again. Four times the trial was postponed. The process dragged on for five agonizing years. The system seemed unconcerned about the wrenching emotions or the fallout from them that affected the doctor, the patient, the respective families, not to mention Sara's other patients, whose care was being serially disrupted by the process.

When the case finally made it to trial, Sara "won." The jury found that she had given appropriate care to Natalie, that she was not responsible for Natalie's actions and subsequent outcome, however tragic. But Sara discovered, like the tens of thousands of doctors who'd been in her shoes, that being exonerated does almost nothing to heal the years of anguish.

Like these tens of thousands of doctors, she realized that the entire system was fundamentally flawed, almost capricious in its malignancy. Lives were nonchalantly destroyed in the process, with little ultimate benefit for patients. Most cases never went to trial, and of those, patients didn't usually win. Even out-of-court settlements rarely settled things sufficiently for anyone. (But the lawyers always benefited financially, no matter what the outcome.)

Unlike these other tens of thousands of doctors, however, Sara decided to do something about it. She spoke to the head of the American Medical Association and the heads of various medical specialty societies and realized that no one was addressing this situation—though almost everyone had a painful malpractice story of his own to tell. The problem was rampant, but, it seemed, it was too painful for anyone to take on.

So Sara began to research the pernicious effects of malpractice on doctors and patients. Additionally, she wrote a book documenting her own malpractice experience.[8] Her extensive interviews and surveys showed that malpractice suits—whether or not they went to trial, irrespective of who won or lost—were soul-corroding events, and that the protracted nature of them ensured maximal pain for all parties involved.[9]

For doctors, the assault on integrity was all-encompassing. Not a single accused doctor emerged unscathed. Even those who knew they had done nothing wrong, even those who were vindicated, suffered wrenching anguish. If it were just bad doctors who were being sued, doctors who practiced substandard medicine or who were arrogant, unfeeling, and uncommunicative, it would be one thing. But just as many suits involved doctors who had long-term, trusting relationships with their patients. Good communication and trust might decrease the number of lawsuits, but it certainly didn't prevent them. Plenty of good and caring doctors found themselves in receipt of one of those dreaded certified letters.[10]

In our interview, Sara told me she'd met a family doctor who delivered a baby with cerebral palsy. The doctor remained close with the family as the primary care doctor for this child and the entire family for twenty years. Right before the child turned twenty-one—just before the statute of limitations expired, that is—the family sued the doctor for malpractice, saying that her medical care during the delivery had led to the cerebral palsy.

The doctor was crushed, astonished that twenty years of close contact, of support and communication, of caring, meant nothing in the end. She could even accept that the family had pursued litigation mainly for financial reasons, out of fear that there wouldn't be resources to care for child after the parents died. Nevertheless, it was demoralizing to the core.

The damage of our malpractice system, however, does not stop at doctors. Ultimately, the most damage may be inflicted upon patients.[11] For the patients involved in lawsuits, this is fairly obvious. The very existence of a suit usually means there was a bad outcome, and the patient is the one who suffers this—regardless of whether the bad outcome was someone's fault or just bad luck. And then to think that your doctor might have delivered inadequate or negligent care feels like a horrible betrayal.

The system itself rarely resolves these feelings (and certainly doesn't undo the bad outcome). The endlessly-dragged-out nature of the legal system is as anguishing to the plaintiff as it is to the defendant. But the fallout extends more broadly to patients, not just to those who have filed malpractice suits. The emotional bruising to doctors caused by the lawsuits profoundly changes these doctors and how they practice medicine. Given that 60 percent or more of doctors eventually get sued, this means that the malevolent effects of malpractice will infiltrate the medical care of the majority of patients. The effects can be substantial; the fact that they may be difficult to isolate makes them even more insidious.

Nearly all sued doctors change how they practice—in ways both large and small—and this can have wide-ranging effects on patients. The tendency toward defensive medicine—overordering tests and treatments—is one of the most common reactions. This may not sound inherently damaging to patients, but in fact it can be harmful, even deadly. Pre-malpractice, a doctor might evaluate a headache with history and physical, then conclude that it's nothing serious and reassure the patient. Post-malpractice, that doctor might not want to risk it and will order a CT scan for every patient with a headache, even if the doctor feels clinically convinced that these headaches do not represent serious disease. Clinical conviction won't hold on the witness stand.

The radiation doses of these extra CT scans add up quickly. It is estimated that radiation from unnecessary CT scans may cause up to three million cases of cancer.[12] (Gilbert Welch's book *Overdiagnosed* is an eye-opening treatise about the harms of excessive testing.)[13] The damage from unnecessary testing is real, and patients are the ones who ultimately suffer.

Then, of course, there's the financial burden. Defensive medicine and liability costs are conservatively estimated to be $55 billion.[14] We can all imagine how much good that money might do if it was directed at, say, malaria prevention, vaccination, or prenatal care.

After experiencing a lawsuit, individual doctors often think twice about whom they treat. Very sick patients, or ones perceived—for whatever reason—to be highly litigious are avoided. After her own lawsuit, Sara Charles stopped treating patients with borderline personality disorder. It wasn't worth the risk. And for these patients, who suffer immensely, there was now one less doctor available.

A survey of orthopedic surgeons revealed that nearly three-quarters avoided medically complex patients in order to minimize lawsuits. Even more tried to stay away from complicated surgeries that carried higher risks of bad outcomes.[15] Multiply this over the tens of thousands of doctors who are bruised from lawsuits, and the result will be that patients with serious medical conditions will find it harder to obtain medical care.

A study of more than seven thousand surgeons found that a quarter had been involved in a recent lawsuit, and that the sued doctors were far more prone to burnout, depression, and suicidal thoughts.[16] The prospect of being operated on by a burned-out, depressed, or suicidal surgeon is rightly terrifying.

Last, there is the effect on doctor-patient connection. This is difficult to measure, but the result can be profound. For the vast majority of physicians who invest their hearts and souls into their work, being accused of malpractice feels like a trust violated. "Physicians do take things personally," Sara Charles wrote in her book, "especially accusations that they have been negligent in their professional practice."[17] These human beings can find it difficult to trust again, for fear of another assault. It is an emotional experience akin to having your spouse cheat on you—and you are very leery about ever trusting again.

Trust is the very basis of a meaningful doctor-patient relationship, and it has to go both ways. When the doctor exudes a hesitancy to trust and invest emotionally, the patient senses this, even if unconsciously. The stage is now set for a wary, suspicious partnership. This doesn't work well in marriages, and it doesn't work well with doctors and patients. It produces just the behavior said to cause lawsuits (and divorces)—poor communication, mistrust, lack of emotional investment.

It is estimated that 75 percent of physicians in low-risk fields (pediatrics, dermatology, psychiatry) will face a lawsuit by the age of sixty-five. For doctors in high-risk fields (neurosurgery, cardiac surgery, obstetrics), it's 99 percent.[18] The way things stand now, the effects of malpractice will reach nearly every patient.

—⁂—

Physicians get judged in a variety of ways; the malpractice suit is only one of them. Within the academic realm of medicine, there is the M & M, where doctors stand before their peers to discuss errors and poor outcomes. Depending on the institution, the atmosphere of M & Ms can range from the emotionally supportive, to the neutrally educational, to the viciously punitive.

These days, doctors are also judged by quality indicators. These are quantitative outcomes—for example, length of hospital stay, percentage of patients with controlled blood pressure—that suggest an objective measure of physician quality. This objectivity, as we will see, is itself prone to subjectivity and bias.

Increasingly, physicians are also judged by patients. This can be done as part of a formal patient-satisfaction survey or on one of a growing number of websites that allow patients to rank their doctors as they do movies and restaurants—one to five stars—and usually include comments about their experiences. More about that later.

There is a school of thought that maintains that being judged is character building and that getting feedback from satisfaction surveys and quality reports is a constructive way to improve. There is certainly some truth to that, but the reality is far more complex and nuanced. Being judged is a double-edged sword, and there are many instances in which the desired practical outcome is smothered by the emotional costs. The fallout for doctors—and their patients—can be staggering.

The quality-measures movement and its sequelae have much in common with the malpractice situation, though the scope and consequences are—for the moment, at least—smaller. The philosophy arose from the idea that there ought to be tangible ways to measure the quality of medical care, that there should be objective ways to distinguish excellent doctors from mediocre ones. Sounds reasonable enough.

The question, of course, is what should be measured? In the case of a general internist or family doctor, possible measurements could be how many of their patients suffer heart attacks, how many quit smoking, how many have cholesterol under 200 and controlled blood pressure, how many have received all appropriate vaccinations.

All of these measures are legitimately part of good health, and doctors would be unanimous in supporting them. But in practice, each of these factors is extremely complicated. Even a relatively straightforward measure, like vaccination rates, depends on a host of variables beyond an individual doctor's quality: number of nurses, coverage by different insurance companies, office-hour flexibility, patient-education level, amount of time allotted per visit, and so on.

This is why so many doctors are uncomfortable with these quality measures. Some have wondered whether these quality measures actually reduce motivation to improve.[19] Selecting out narrow data points to measure may work well for assembly-line type work, but it can be counterproductive for complex tasks that involve deliberation, decision-making, judgment, communication, and creativity.[20] Focusing on the minutiae—even if those are individually important measurements—can undermine a person's desire and ability to improve. (Offering more control over one's work environment and improving overall job satisfaction seems to do a better job.)

My own experience in being evaluated for "quality" left me with that same horrible feeling about being judged. Our hospital had undertaken a laudable and Herculean effort to improve the care of patients with diabetes. There was no disagreement that diabetes was one of the most complicated diseases we faced and that these patients would benefit from the best medical care possible.

In that light, each doctor was given a report card citing the percentage of his or her patients whose glucose, blood pressure, and cholesterol were at goal. These seemed like reasonable data points to evaluate how good a job we were doing.

My report card was dismal, way below the targets our institution had set. It made me feel awful, because I was putting everything I had into my job. But I felt guilty about the bad numbers, so I worked harder, staying later in the office and calling patients from home on evenings and weekends. Still, my numbers didn't seem to budge; it was downright dispiriting.

I wrote about this experience for both the *New England Journal of Medicine* and the *New York Times.*[21] In those essays, I tried to point out that these sorts of metrics don't give a full measure of quality; they simply measure what is easy for administrators to measure but do not necessarily add up to the totality of good medical care.

The responses were swift and vehement. "Dr. Ofri, are you afraid to be measured by hard data?" was the common refrain.

Well . . . yes. I was. It was just like sitting with those lawyers again, having my every utterance and action scrutinized. Once again under the bright lights with unsmiling observers just waiting to find my flaws and broadcast them to the world.

In my articles, I focused on the problems of quality measures, how, like the blind men touching the elephant, they describe only isolated parts of a medical encounter. I pointed out that when they need a doctor, most people—including doctors themselves—ask for personal recommendations about someone who is smart, caring, thorough, thoughtful, and trustworthy, not someone with the best stats.

I pounded away at the concrete problems with quality measures, but the truth was that what was driving me to write so much about this was the horrific discomfort of being judged, about the possibility that some "objective" body could destroy what my heart, soul, and life were committed to. I knew that this was largely an emotional response, but I couldn't escape it.

—⟋⟋⟍—

And then there are the evaluations of physicians by patients. Patients have always shared information about doctors via word of mouth. In fact, as I've noted, this is the way most people find their doctors. The Internet and social-networking sites have now taken this to a new level, so instead of hearing recommendations from just friends and neighbors, you can get the lowdown from the larger online community.

I remember the moment when a local rating site that had previously limited itself to household services started rating physicians. They ran ads on our public radio station, and so every hour on the hour, I would hear: "Angie's List—rating plumbers, cleaning services . . . *and now doctors too!*" I couldn't help but notice the note of triumph in the emphasis: *and now doctors too!* It was as if it were saying, *We gotcha now, you crafty doctors, trying to sneak around unrated!*

The number of rating sites has proliferated briskly, even faster, it seems, than drug-resistant staph in an ICU. The typical Internet search on a doctor yields only rating sites for the first few pages. You have to scroll quite a ways before you find actual information about that doctor—bio, hospital affiliation, practice website, professional memberships, board certification.

And just as brisk has been the development of the online-reputation managers, many of which target physicians. Doctors—who stand to lose greatly from bad reviews, and who presumably have more money and less time than average joes—are an appealing target. At the rate this is going, every doctor will be required to have a personal online-reputation manager along with the standard malpractice insurance.

There are many who feel that choosing one's doctor should require slightly more sophisticated thinking than choosing a toaster oven or a Mexican restaurant. But a growing number of people feel that patient ratings are indispensable for getting a fuller sense of a doctor's qualifications, something beyond the standard listing of license, board certification, and office hours.

Unsurprisingly, doctors have not warmed to this as much as patients have. Doctors worry that patients who are annoyed over small slights (being kept waiting too long) or things out of the doctor's control (insurance issues) will vent with vindictive comments that can easily ruin a reputation. Because most doctors receive only a handful of ratings each—many fewer than local Chinese take-outs—one or two negative reviews can exert outsize influence. The fact that most users are anonymous and aren't required to register anywhere raises the possibility of easy vendettas (though there are a few sites that do require registration). There is no way to verify that the users have actually even been seen by a particular physician.

These reviews often end up focusing on the externalities of care, such as how nice the doctor is or how friendly the office staff are or how many tests are ordered—things that are readily observable to anyone. But can they evaluate how up to date the doctor is or how good the actual medical care is?

I've never been one to spend time digging around the Internet for these sorts of personal reviews—it has always seemed so sordid and gossipy—but I felt that I needed to obtain primary data for this book. And so I waded in—strictly for research purposes, of course. As I began browsing around, I started seeing ratings of colleagues I worked with, former students and residents I'd trained, even my own doctors. The voyeuristic impulse set in immediately. I wanted to see what patients were writing about people I knew, but it felt awkward, especially when I stumbled across negative comments.

I came upon the ratings of a doctor I knew as a colleague but also used as a physician for myself. What I liked about her was her no-nonsense approach to both medicine and life. She believed in being honest, without any sugarcoating. This is a personality style that appeals to some people but might turn others off, and this was apparent in her ratings. Half the patients gave her five stars, saying, "She is great! I love her! Would definitely recommend her." The other half gave her one star, with comments like "I would not recommend this Doctor to my worst enemies. Period!!!!!" They gave everything about her the lowest rating, even her medical knowledge and clinical skills.

Having been her patient, I knew that she was blunt, and I could see how this style might come across as abrasive to some, but there was nothing slipshod in her practice of medicine. And knowing her collegially gave me insight into her commitment to medicine; she always talked about her practice with enthusiasm and love. But it seemed that patients who didn't like her style of communicating generalized their feelings to every aspect of her medical practice.

This points back, of course, to how our emotional responses color everything we see. But more broadly, it shows how hard it can be to deliver meaningful appraisals. Doddering doctors with rich bedside manners but skills that haven't been updated in half a century might garner higher ratings than diagnostic geniuses with Neanderthal interpersonal skills (the real-life Gregory Houses of the world). This is not to say that bedside manner is more or less important than clinical skills, but these doctor-rating sites suffer from as many limitations as the supposedly objective quality measures.

I felt terrible seeing harsh reviews for this doctor whom I knew to be competent and committed and in whose care I'd felt assured and safe. It seemed like a supreme injustice. There were rotten doctors out there deserving of these reviews, but not her. Who would be left if we drove out the good doctors? I decided that I needed to add my own positive assessment to counter some of the excessively negative ones. It was odd to participate in a system that I have mixed feelings about, but I nevertheless typed in my five-star recommendation, adding in a surfeit of exclamation points that would have made my high-school English teacher blanch.

With some trepidation, I decided to check myself out on these ratings sites. After all, it was for research purposes. My first impression was shock at how much these sites knew about me. I've never had any contact with them, but they had quite a bit to offer up on me. First off, each site was sure to state my age and how many years since I'd graduated medical school. I realize that this is easily accessible information, but still, having one's age printed there, front and center, felt sort of personal—the kind of thing I might omit on a professional résumé. In fact, it turns out that personal information about physicians is relatively common on the web.[22]

There were all sorts of oddities associated with me on these sites, things I certainly hadn't put out there. One site suggested to patients that before they visit Dr. Ofri, they ought to read "8 Ways to Manage Hemorrhoids." But at least my height, weight, and penchant for clunky shoes weren't listed.

In the end, I wasn't able to find any comments about me as a doctor. I'd like to think that this was a ringing endorsement of my medical abilities, but it was more likely because most of my patients lack the financial, educational, and linguistic resources to post online reviews. The experience actually left me a little sad, because it was a reminder of the obstacles my patients face. But I confess that it was also a relief. Some of the reviews of doctors were scathing, and if my patients thought that of me, it would be more than I could bear.

—⁂—

Mercedes's mysterious death—one of my most devastating cases ever—turned out to be its own form of judgment. Though her case never went to trial, it never felt entirely settled to me. *Something* killed her, and we never learned what.

Two weeks after Mercedes died, my medical residency finished. I walked out of the hospital with half a notion never to return. What should have been the crowning moment at the end of a decade's worth of medical school, scientific research, and residency was instead a moment of splintering doubt.

Until then, I had been steeped in a medical culture in which knowledge was equated with power. The more we knew, the better doctors we'd be. We crammed knowledge down our throats, like geese in the French countryside being force-fed for foie gras. For ten solid years I'd barely come up for air, because I knew that I needed this knowledge.

But Mercedes's death was a clean slap in the face, a direct hit to the foundations that I'd built for myself as a fledgling doctor. If all the collective knowledge of my colleagues, my attendings, my journals, my books, my library searches could wither helplessly as a beautiful twenty-three-year-old woman died in front of my eyes, then what exactly was I doing as a doctor? This self-judgment was more harrowing than anything the lawyers could have dealt out.

While the rest of my residency colleagues started fellowships or jobs the minute residency ended, I chose to cut myself off from the hospital world. While my friends established themselves as independent doctors or trained further to become cardiologists or nephrologists, I roamed the small towns of Guatemala and Mexico studying Spanish and catching up on a decade's worth of missed novels. I supported myself with one-month stints as a temp doc here and there, but I stayed clear of the intense world of academic medicine. I needed to think. And perhaps even more, I needed to feel.

I spent eighteen months on the road, trawling the Central and South American countrysides where so many of my patients hailed from. I hadn't met Julia at that point, but my travels took me within a crow's flight of her village. It was during these wanderings that I began to write about my experiences with patients, including Mercedes. The deliberate pace of writing—in stark contrast to the breakneck speed of medicine—allowed me time to revisit these experiences. It gave me space for the deeper consideration I felt my patients deserved, something that was simply impossible in the real time of medicine.

While bunking in the youth hostels of Guatemala, I wrote down everything I could remember about Mercedes. I spent months working on her story—revising, rethinking, reliving. It eventually formed the ending of my first book, *Singular Intimacies: Becoming a Doctor at Bellevue.*

And while I was intellectually frustrated, I felt strangely emotionally complete. That night in the ICU with Mercedes was excruciatingly painful, but it was also perhaps my most authentic experience as a doctor. Something was sad. And I cried. Simple logic, but so rarely adhered to in the high-octane world of academic medicine. Standing in the ICU, the chaplain's arms around me, surrounded by Mercedes's family, I felt like a person. Not like a physician or a scientist or an emissary from the world of rational logic, but just a person. Like each of the other persons who were locked in that tight circle around Bed 10. There was a strength in that circle that I'd never felt from my colleagues or my professors. A strength that allowed me to release the tense determination for intellectual mastery that had so supported me as a doctor. After years of honing those muscles, it was a deliriously aching relief to let them go.

And it didn't turn me away from medicine; it enticed me. I did need a break, but I knew that I would come back. I still wanted to learn more and become a smarter doctor, but I also wanted to be in this world populated with living, breathing, feeling people. I wanted to be in this sacred zone that was alive with real feelings, theirs and mine. I still didn't know why I had initially entered the field of medicine ten years ago, but I now knew why I wanted to stay.[23]

Julia, part seven

Forty-eight hours after Julia entered the operating room in Columbia University to receive her heart transplant, I set off for two weeks' worth of lectures. Frankly, it was the last thing I wanted to do at that moment, but these lectures had been planned nearly a year in advance. And I knew that Julia was in good hands.

And if I was truly honest with myself, I knew that I didn't have a medical role at this moment. I was her primary care doctor, so my job was to take care of her general health, help her manage her complex cardiac disease, remember her flu shots and medication refills—to keep her alive, really, until a heart transplant could become available. And now it had, so it was appropriate for me to step aside and let the transplant specialists and cardiologists handle this phase. There was no need to add more cooks to this already complicated broth. I'd be ready for her at the Bellevue Medical Clinic when her normal life was ready to resume.

And what a pleasure it would be to return to the mundane side of medicine. How blissful it would be to order a mammogram or a Pap smear, screening tests that, by definition, posit a future. The very act of worrying about diseases that are yet to come implies that there is a yet to come. For so long, I'd been too frightened to permit myself to even contemplate a "yet to come" for Julia. But now, we at least had a chance.

I didn't kid myself, however, that the next year or two would be a cakewalk. On the contrary, I was fully cognizant of the burdens of the immunosuppressive medications that Julia would be required to take for the rest of her life. I had seen a few patients through this process and it was never easy. The first six months would be the roughest.

Rejection was an ever-present worry. Complications from those highly toxic meds were no small matter. I wouldn't be a Pollyanna about the challenges that Julia still faced, but at least there was something to face. I zigzagged from Boston to Dallas to Rochester to Baltimore, stopping home for a day or two and then taking off again. Back-to-back lectures were not my preference, but somehow this particular October had accumulated so many commitments. I would be glad when it was all over.

I stayed in contact with the cardiologists at Columbia and kept tabs on Julia's progress. As expected, her healthy body tided her through the arduous surgery. Nothing, of course, is ever textbook when transplanting an organ from one body to another, but Julia was doing satisfactorily, and plans were proceeding for discharge to cardiac rehab.

I traveled from lecture to lecture on a sustained high. I had been using sections of my book *Medicine in Translation* to talk about how doctors work with patients from different cultures. I frequently read aloud parts about Julia during my lectures to highlight the challenges of immigration status, of language, of traumatic history. But now I had a happy ending to add. So many of the medical stories that I weave into my lectures have tragic endings, so this felt like a singular moment—literarily and medically. I was brimming with faith in medicine, faith in humanity. I preached the gospel so enthusiastically at one lecture that I was sure the audience of hospital administrators would drop every last spreadsheet and begin cramming organic chemistry so they could take the MCATs.

That Tuesday afternoon found me sitting outdoors with my laptop in the taxi pick-up area of a hotel parking lot in Baltimore, taking advantage of the free WiFi that extended from the lobby. It wasn't the most pleasant locale, given the fumes from the taxis, the cigarette smoke from the drivers, and the incessant honking. But it was better than the lobby, whose high-volume, top-forty Muzak made any semblance of coherent thought impossible.

I was sorting through e-mails amid the grittiness when the terse message arrived from the cardiologist: Julia had suffered two strokes.

The python of anxiety that had accompanied me all during those years with Julia, that had been triumphantly vanquished ten days ago, resurrected itself with a rapidity and a rabidity that froze every last nerve. Strokes? I was flooded with frantic questions: Big strokes? Little strokes? Hemorrhagic? Embolic? The kind from which you recover? The kind that paralyze you? The python constricted as the possibilities fanned themselves out with grim precision.

I scrambled for more information but felt like my mind was swimming through mud, the phrase that Julia had used to describe her body in the absence of an adequate blood supply. My neurons plodded in agonizingly slow motion as I struggled to piece together what was happening two hundred miles away from this parking lot.

A frenzied medical evaluation had ensued in the transplant unit: What had caused the strokes? Was it reversible? Could medications temper the effects? The neurosurgeons went so far as to drill a burr hole in her skull to biopsy her brain tissue, in the hope that an infection might be found, something treatable.

But in the end it was determined that Julia's brain and vasculature, so accustomed to the limp dribbles of blood from her battered heart, was simply overwhelmed by the vigorous salvos of a robust, twenty-two-year-old heart.

As I sat there on the parking-lot bench, frozen in the grip of this inner python, the next message arrived: life support will be withdrawn.

I read and reread those words: life . . . support . . . will . . . be . . . withdrawn. My eyes scraped back and forth along the phrase, chafing against the cruel, passive construction.

Life support will be withdrawn.

The honking taxis and the diesel fumes faded away. The exhilaration of the transplant news melted like wax. The heroic administrative efforts of the Bellevue staff evanesced. Julia's quiet fortitude during her many hospitalizations seeped silently away. Tears slid down my cheeks as the layers of Julia's life seemed to wick away from my grasp until I was left empty-handed.

It seemed impossible that this was happening. We had been so close. It had been roughly three thousand days since I'd stood in Julia's room on the 16-West ward of Bellevue Hospital, defeated in my efforts to enunciate her death sentence. Three thousand days in a medical and emotional labyrinth, taunted the entire way by the cruel contradictions of circumstance. Three thousand days, but we'd arrived. Somehow, Julia had survived and clawed her way forward. When the good fortune of the transplant arrived, it seemed like divine justice. And then, like an anvil, fate slammed us down.

We had been so close!

—⁓—

The next morning I boarded an Amtrak train bound for New York. The people and conversations that jostled around me converged into a generalized sensory sludge. I stared out the window but caught little of the East Coast scenery that spooled listlessly by. The train chugged northward, the chalky sensation in my gut growing heavier and grainier with each passing mile. There is nothing pure or noble about grief, despite how my favorite novels and operas depict it. Just muck.

At Penn Station, instead of hopping into my usual crosstown taxi home, I lugged my suitcase through the subway turnstile and boarded an A train. The subway rattled uptown, 150 miserable jarring blocks toward the Columbia University Hospital.

Inside the hospital, I wandered the halls for a good twenty minutes. I was too out of sorts to ask directions, preferring to traipse around till I found the ICU on my own. Julia was alone when I finally located her; her family had gone for lunch. She was propped up in the bed, eyes closed, preternaturally still. Her hair was longer than I recalled it, thicker and blacker. The locks stood out in their dense luster against the white sheets and baby-blue hospital gown. As I drew closer and noticed the bangs oddly askew, I realized that it was a wig. Her head must have been shaved for the brain biopsy.

I squeezed myself, my coat, and my suitcase into the narrow ICU room, wedging into the cramped space between Julia's bed and the armada of monitors. The breathing tube had been removed, and she was breathing on her own, though shallowly. For the moment she looked as though she were sleeping peacefully, but I knew that it was just a matter of time. The intracranial swelling from the massive strokes would inexorably obliterate the brainstem structures responsible for respiration and heartbeats. I closed my eyes and took a breath to settle myself, but the air chafed in my throat. Reluctantly, I pulled my eyes open to face what I did not want to see.

It really was Julia. The Julia who had journeyed thousands of miles, the Julia who had faced more adversity than any human should ever bear, the Julia who possessed a fortitude that was both staggering and understated, the Julia who was now being slowly, excruciatingly vanquished by this life.

I reached over and took Julia's hand in mine. It was limp, but warm. Bruises and scabs from a cavalcade of recent IVs littered her forearm. I stroked the paper-thin skin and glanced at her nails—neatly filed and polished, probably by her sister. There was so much I wanted to say to Julia, but I didn't know how to begin. Something in me wanted to start at the beginning and trace the whole story with her, recount as much of her life as I knew.

But each time I started, my words petered out after a line or two. There is only so much conversation, even monologue, that you can have with a comatose person. To have your words hanging in the air, unanswered, unregistered, unmoored, is disorienting and feels too self-conscious. Everything I said felt trite and awkward.

Then an idea came to me. I couldn't converse with her, but perhaps I could read to her. In my suitcase was my marked-up copy of *Medicine in Translation*. I didn't carry it with me on a regular basis; it was with me only because I'd happened to come to the hospital straight from my lecture in Baltimore. I tugged it out and flipped to page 28, where I'd marked several passages with pencil.

"Julia is a thirty-six-year-old Guatemalan female with an exacerbation of congestive heart failure," began chapter 4.

While Julia lay in bed, unmoving, seemingly restful, I recounted how the intern first presented her case to me. Reading aloud to Julia felt natural somehow, even though I knew that she would not be able to hear me in any conscious sense. Something about tracing the narrative of her life seemed like the right thing to offer at this closing moment. It was the only thing, really.

I reconstructed our first meeting, my inability to tell Julia the full truth about her diagnosis. The ICU hummed around us with a quiet busyness, but no one disturbed us as I turned the pages, tracing the three thousand days across which our lives had intersected.

There was the time she'd given me a hand-knitted cap for my new baby. There was a five-dollar bill folded inside, which she would not permit me to decline.

There was the time she'd been trying desperately to get Vasco, her son, out of the detention center in Texas but wasn't strong enough to travel there. We'd worked together on the letter I wrote on her behalf, trying to make clear the gravity of her illness without making her seem too sick to care for her son.

There was the time I told her about my trip to Tikal, the famous Mayan ruins in northern Guatemala. It was only two hundred miles from the town of her birth, roughly the same distance from Baltimore to New York, but she'd never been able to visit—and now never would. It fell to her gringo doctor to describe it to her during one of our medical appointments, in embarrassingly error-laden Spanish.

There were the conversations with the cardiology fellow, trying to figure out how to beat the odds and get her on the transplant list.

And then, of course, there was the day she showed up to clinic in the snowstorm, having resurrected herself from the weeks near death in the ICU. It seemed like a miracle at the time.

It was nearly a half an hour before I reached the end of the story, at least the end that I had written. I closed the book and then folded my hands over hers, resting my forehead on the railing of her bed. The final chapter of Julia's story had ineluctably arrived, and we were dwelling in its exact calyx. It would be another week before I paid my final, formal respects at the storefront funeral home in Brooklyn. Julia would be wearing a white satin gown—her wedding dress, perhaps—and the wig would be more precisely arranged. But her hands would be cold when I held them, with a bleak, unsettling solidity about them.

For now, though, her hands retained the pliancy of life, however tenuous in actual, biological terms. I wanted to hold on as long as I could, to stay enmeshed within the exquisite yielding of skin against skin.

We sat that way, soundlessly, for what felt like an eon of grief. At some point, I had run out of tears, but still I couldn't bring myself to leave. We'd said good-bye to each other hundreds of times over the years. At each one, I'd worried that it would be our last. Now we'd actually reached it. The last good-bye.

And what does one actually do in a final good-bye? Would I simply just say that— "Good-bye"? Would I shake her hand? Give her a kiss? A hug? All these protocols of parting seemed strained. All of these required the Julia that I knew, who would respond with a distinctly human rejoinder. Without that, these actions felt hollow, absurd.

Out of the corner of my eye, I caught sight of a burgundy stethoscope dangling from the cardiac monitor, a cheap one, the kind just for taking blood pressure. But the reflex was automatic. I yanked it down and snapped in the earpieces. The metal bell of a stranger's stethoscope nestled itself between the second and third fingers of my right hand.

Just as I'd done countless times over the years, I slipped the flat diaphragm of the stethoscope through the opening of Julia's gown. Without my even having to direct it, the metal disk settled into the comfortable parasternal concavity where I always begin my cardiac exams.

Feeling unrushed and oddly at ease, I glided the diaphragm along the familiar planes of the heart, pausing at the aortic, pulmonic, tricuspid, and mitral landmarks. I dwelled longer at each spot than I normally did, as though compelled to bid farewell to each voice in the quartet.

This heart sounded different, of course, lacking the systolic murmurs whose auditory curvature I knew so intimately. But it was still Julia's heart, beating mournfully along the decrescendo of her life.

"The final common pathway is the heart," John Stone wrote in his poem "Gaudeamus Igitur." "For what matters finally is how the human spirit is spent."[1] I eased the bell out from under the material and carefully retied the gown. Then I draped the stethoscope back over the cardiac monitor and turned to gaze at her one last time. Despite the hardships of her life, Julia had maintained an uncanny tenderness, enduring but also prospering, savoring a life filled with love.

Her human spirit had indeed been well spent.

Afterword

The doctor-patient interaction is fundamentally a human connection, and emotions are a de facto part of it. The goal of this book has been to attune both doctors and patients to the emotional *basso continuo* of this interaction. For doctors—especially for those in training—it is critical to be aware of the potent influence of emotion on our "rational" decision making. Remaining cognizant of our emotions, being attuned to their fluctuations, understanding how best to integrate them in the moment of connection with a patient will offer the patient the most solid and trusting setting.

For patients—and all of us doctors are of course patients at one time or another—it is one more tool for maximizing the quality of medical care. Keeping your inner ear open to the emotional subtext—both yours and your doctor's—can help keep the focus on what is most important. "Patients . . . swim together with physicians in a sea of feelings," writes Jerome Groopman. "Each needs to keep an eye on a neutral shore where flags are planted to warn of perilous emotional currents."

The shore isn't always neutral, despite our desire for it to be so, despite Osler's insistence on *equanimitas*. Recognizing both the sea and the shore is essential. In this book, I've focused mainly on emotions that are often called negative—fear, shame, grief, anger, being overwhelmed—because these are the ones that exert the strongest influence on medical care. But I'm fully aware of the spectrum of positive emotions that exist in medicine—joy, pride, gratitude, even love. These can certainly affect the care that patients receive. Usually these exert positive influences on medical care—doctors who find joy in their work usually do a better job than doctors who are angry, ashamed, or burned out. But even positive emotions have the potential for negative influences. A classic example is doctors who care for friends or family members. The closeness and love can inhibit the doctor from asking awkward questions or doing uncomfortable procedures—asking about sexual history, performing a rectal exam, or questioning drug use, for example.

I chose the story of Julia to weave throughout this book because of the profound and lasting effects she had on me. Besides the roller coaster of medical travails that marked our years together, we also experienced just about every emotion in the dictionary. There were moments of pride, gratitude, humor, and affection. There was fear, anxiety, guilt, and foreboding. I've never had a more joyous moment in my medical career as when that new heart was sewn inside her. And I've never been more grief-stricken than when it all came crashing down. Even now, years later, when I write about that moment, I need to pause to allow the rekindled grief to settle itself back down. I have shared Julia's story to honor her memory and also to portray how emotions infuse and affect the doctor-patient interaction at every level.

—m—

Doctors often don't get the distinction between curing and healing, but patients instinctively do. For most doctors, if the disease has been eradicated—well, that's success. For patients, that's only part of the process—a significant one, obviously, but not the only one. Plenty of patients walk out of our hospitals, clinics, and offices with their diseases under control, and yet they do not feel healed.

Paying attention to emotions within the doctor-patient interaction doesn't guarantee healing, no doubt. But ignoring them surely makes it less likely. "Healing is a matter of time," wrote Hippocrates, "but it is sometimes also a matter of opportunity."[1] Taking this opportunity can be prescriptive for both doctors and patients.

—∽∾—

Thirty-six years after Dr. Osler's "Aequanimitas" speech, Dr. Francis Peabody gave another commencement address to another graduating class of eager medical students. He summed up his ideas in this now famous phrase: "The secret of the care of the patient is in caring for the patient."[2] In this deceptively simple axiom, he encompassed compassion, empathy, and human connection, along with all the medical technologies and therapeutic modalities that a doctor can offer to a patient. Beyond curing, this is what offers the possibility of healing.

Acknowledgments

A book about doctors and patients owes its primary gratitude to the doctors and patients whose stories form the basis of the book. Curtis Climer, Sara Charles, Herdley Paolini, "Eva," and "Joanne" all spent hours of their time talking with me and sharing their stories, in many cases some of their deepest and most painful recollections. I am indebted to their patients and to my patients for leaving indelible impressions and imparting valuable lessons that will help future patients.

There were many doctors and patients who gave generously of their time but whose stories did not end up in the limited pages available. I am equally grateful to them, as well as to my Bellevue colleagues who shared anecdotes, advice, and encouragement along the way.

For literary and topical inspiration, I give thanks to Drs. Oliver Sacks, Jerome Groopman, Abraham Verghese, Rafael Campo, Richard Selzer, Sherwin Nuland, and Perri Klass, whose sage writings and thoughtful approaches to patient care have been models for me. I've never quite gotten over the death of Dr. John Stone and try my best to quote him in every lecture I give. Very few people can achieve the trifecta of being a genteel Southerner, a top-flight cardiologist, and a wise poet all at once.

Several parts of this book have appeared in journals and newspapers. I am particularly grateful to the *New York Times* editors Toby Bilanow, Honor Jones, David Corcoran, and Mary Giordano. Many thanks to Ellen Ficklen and her team at *Health Affairs*. The editors of the *New England Journal of Medicine*, especially Deborah Malina, have been stalwart supporters throughout my writing career.

The heavy-lifting award for this book goes to Beacon Press. Helene Atwan is an editor nonpareil, who manages to find time for hours-long phone conversations to assuage every last author neurosis. Beacon is a remarkable and dedicated publishing house, and I am indebted to Tom Hallock, Pam MacColl, Crystal Paul, Marcy Barnes, Bob Kosturko, Susan Lumenello, and all the staff that keep independent publishing alive and flourishing.

Starting a new book project is like stepping into a new world, and it can be even more fun if you actually do step off into a new world while writing, especially with your best friend. Thank you, Benjy, for embarking on our year-long adventure in Israel, and for your endless support and love.

I've always fantasized of living the Zen writing life—serene, orderly, meditative. Luckily, I have my Naava, Noah, and Ariel to ensure that I never transgress into any such malarkey.

Notes

INTRODUCTION

1. Jerome Groopman, *How Doctors Think* (Boston: Houghton Mifflin, 2007), 40.
2. M. C. McConnell and K. Eva, "The Role of Emotion in the Learning and Transfer of Clinical Skills and Knowledge," *Academic Medicine* 87 (2012): 1316–22.
3. Antonio Damasio, *Looking for Spinoza: Joy, Sorrow, and the Feeling Brain* (New York: Harcourt, 2003), 3.
4. William Osler, "Aequanimitas," speech, *Celebrating the Contributions of William Osler*, website, Johns Hopkins University, http://www.medicalarchives .jhmi.edu/.
5. Groopman, *How Doctors Think*, 39.

JULIA, PART ONE

1. Danielle Ofri, "Doctors Have Feelings Too," *New York Times*, March 28, 2012.

CHAPTER TWO

1. Alessio Avenanti, Angela Sirigu, and Salvatore M. Aglioti, "Racial Bias Reduces Empathic Sensorimotor Resonance with Other-Race Pain," *Current Biology* (2010): 1018–22.
2. B. W. Newton et al., "Is There Hardening of the Heart During Medical School?" *Academic Medicine* 83 (2008): 244–49; M. Hojat et al., "The Devil Is in the Third Year: A Longitudinal Study of Erosion of Empathy in Medical School," *Academic Medicine* 84 (2009): 1182–91; M. Neumann et al., "Empathy Decline and Its Reasons: A Systematic Review of Studies with Medical Students and Residents," *Academic Medicine* 86 (2011): 996–1009.
3. D. Wear et al., "Making Fun of Patients: Medical Students' Perceptions and Use of Derogatory and Cynical Humor in Clinical Settings," *Academic Medicine* 81 (2006): 454–62; G. N. Parsons et al., "Between Two Worlds," *Journal of General Internal Medicine* 16 (2001): 544–49; D. Wear et al., "Derogatory and Cynical Humour Directed Towards Patients: Views of Residents and Attending Doctors," *Medical Education* 43 (2009): 34–41.
4. M. Hojat et al., "The Jefferson Scale of Physician Empathy: Development and Preliminary Psychometric Data," *Educational and Psychological Measurement* 61 (2001): 349–65.
5. M. Hojat, *Empathy in Patient Care: Antecedents, Development, Measurement, and Outcomes* (New York: Springer, 2006).
6. M. Hojat et al., "Empathy in Medical Students As Related to Academic Performance, Clinical Competence, and Gender," *Medical Education* 36 (2002): 1–6;

S. Gonnella et al., "Empathy Scores in Medical School and Ratings of Empathic Behavior in Residency Training Three Years Later," *Journal of Social Psychology* 145 (2005): 663–72; M. Hojat et al., "The Jefferson Scale of Physician Empathy: Further Psychometric Data and Differences by Gender and Specialty at Item Level," *Academic Medicine* 77 (2002), S58–S60; M. Hojat et al., "Patient Perceptions of Physician Empathy, Satisfaction with Physician, Interpersonal Trust, and Compliance," *International Journal of Medical Education* 1 (2010): 83–88.

7. S. Rosenthal et al., "Preserving Empathy in Third-Year Medical Students," *Academic Medicine* 86 (2011): 350–58.

8. D. A. Christakis and C. Feudtner, "Temporary Matters: The Ethical Consequences of Transient Social Relationships in Medical Training," *Journal of the American Medical Association* 278 (1997): 739–43.

9. D. Hirsh et al., "Educational Outcomes of the Harvard Medical School–Cambridge Integrated Clerkship: A Way Forward for Medical Education," *Academic Medicine* 87 (2012): 643–50.

10. "Preliminary Recommendations," *MR5: 5th Comprehensive Review of the Medical College Admission Test (MCAT)*, American Association of Medical Colleges, https://www.aamc.org/.

11. J. Coulehan et al., "'Let Me See If I Have This Right . . .': Words That Build Empathy," *Annals of Internal Medicine* 135 (2001): 221–27.

12. M. Hojat et al., "Physicians' Empathy and Clinical Outcomes in Diabetic Patients," *Academic Medicine* 86 (2011): 359–64.

13. S. S. Kim, S. Kaplowitz, and M. V. Johnston, "The Effects of Physician Empathy on Patient Satisfaction and Compliance," *Evaluation and the Health Professions* 27 (2004): 237–51.

14. M. Neumann et al., "Determinants and Patient-Reported Long-Term Outcomes of Physician Empathy in Oncology: A Structural Equation Modeling Approach," *Patient Education and Counseling* 69 (2007): 63–75.

15. D. P. Rakel et al., "Practitioner Empathy and the Duration of the Common Cold," *Family Medicine* 41 (2009): 494–501.

16. S. Del Canale et al., "The Relationship Between Physician Empathy and Disease Complications: An Empirical Study of Primary Care Physicians and Their Diabetic Patients in Parma, Italy," *Academic Medicine* 87 (2012): 1243–49.

JULIA, PART TWO

1. Danielle Ofri, *Medicine in Translation: Journeys with My Patients* (Boston: Beacon Press, 2010), 224.

CHAPTER 3

1. J. LeDoux, "The Amygdala," *Current Biology* 17 (2007): 868–74.

2. J. S. Feinstein et al., "The Human Amygdala and the Induction and Experience of Fear," *Current Biology* 21 (2011): 34–38.

3. Ernest Becker, *The Denial of Death* (New York: Free Press, 1973).

4. L. N. Dyrbye et al., "Systematic Review of Depression, Anxiety, and Other Indicators of Psychological Distress Among U.S. and Canadian Medical Students," *Academic Medicine* 81 (2006): 354–73.

5. V. R. LeBlanc, "The Effects of Acute Stress on Performance: Implications for Health Professions Education," *Academic Medicine* 84 (2009): S25–S33.

6. J. S. Lerner and D. Keltner, "Fear, Anger, and Risk," *Journal of Personality and Social Psychology* 81 (2001): 146–59.

7. A. C. Miu et al., "Anxiety Impairs Decision-Making: Psychophysiological Evidence from an Iowa Gambling Task," *Biological Psychology* 77 (2008): 353–58.

8. J. D. McCue and C. L. Sachs, "A Stress Management Workshop Improves Residents' Coping Skills," *Archives of Internal Medicine* 151 (1991): 2273–77; Support Groups: C. Ghetti et al., "Burnout, Psychological Skills, and Empathy: Balint Training in Obstetrics and Gynecology Residents," *Journal of Graduate Medical Education* (2009): 231–35; Mindfulness Meditation: M. S. Krasner et al., "Association of an Educational Program in Mindful Communication with Burnout, Empathy, and Attitudes Among Primary Care Physicians," *Journal of the American Medical Association* 302 (2009): 1284–93.

9. A. P. Smith and M. Woods, "Effects of Chewing Gum on the Stress and Work of University Students," *Appetite* 58 (2012): 1037–40.

10. J. M. Milstein et al., "Burnout Assessment in House Officers: Evaluation of an Intervention to Reduce Stress," *Medical Teacher* 31 (2009): 338–41.

11. I. Christakis, "Measuring the Stress of the Surgeons in Training and Use of a Novel Interventional Program to Combat It," *Journal of the Korean Surgical Society* 82 (2012): 312–16.

12. E. R. Stucky et al., "Intern to Attending: Assessing Stress Among Physicians," *Academic Medicine* 84 (2009): 251–57; I. Ahmed, "Cognitive Emotions: Depression and Anxiety in Medical Students and Staff," *Journal of Critical Care* 24 (2009): e1–e18.

13. Danielle Ofri, "A Difficult Patient's Journey," review of *My Imaginary Illness*, *Lancet* 377 (2011): 2074.

14. Danielle Ofri, "Drowning in a Sea of Health Complaints," *New York Times*, February 11, 2011, http://well.blogs.nytimes.com/.

15. Jerome Groopman, *How Doctors Think* (Boston: Houghton Mifflin, 2007).

16. K. G. Shojania et al., "Changes in Rates of Autopsy-Detected Diagnostic Errors over Time," *Journal of the American Medical Association* 289 (2003): 2849–56; L. Goldman et al., "The Value of the Autopsy in Three Different Eras" *New England Journal of Medicine* 308 (1983): 1000–1005; M. L. Graber, "Diagnostic Error in Internal Medicine," *Archives of Internal Medicine* 165 (2005): 1493–99.

17. G. R. Norman and K. W. Eva, "Diagnostic Error and Clinical Reasoning," *Medical Education* 44 (2010): 94–100.

CHAPTER 4

1. L. Granek et al., "Nature and Impact of Grief Over Patient Loss on Oncologists' Personal and Professional Lives," *Archives of Internal Medicine* 172 (2012): 964–66.

2. M. Shayne and T. Quill, "Oncologists Responding to Grief," *Archives of Internal Medicine* 172 (2012): 966–67.

3. Danielle Ofri, "A Patient, a Death, but No One to Grieve," *New York Times*, May 17, 2010.

CHAPTER 5

1. Aaron Lazare, *On Apology* (New York: Oxford University Press, 2004).

2. D. W. Winnicott, "Transitional Objects and Transitional Phenomena: A Study of the First Not-Me Possession," *International Journal of Psychoanalysis* 34 (1953): 89–97.

3. M. E. Collins et al., "On the Prospects for a Blame-Free Medical Culture," *Social Science and Medicine* 69 (2009): 1287–90.

4. Ibid.

5. U. H. Lindstrom et al., "Medical Students' Experiences of Shame in Professional Enculturation," *Medical Education* 45 (2011): 1016–24.

6. Lazare, *Apology*, 168.

7. Collins, "On the Prospects."

8. W. Cunningham and S. Dovey, "The Effect on Medical Practice of Disciplinary Complaints: Potentially Negative for Patient Care," *New Zealand Medical Journal* 113 (2000): 464–67.

9. A. W. Wu et al., "Do House Officers Learn from Their Mistakes?" *Journal of the American Medical Association* 265 (1991): 2089–94.

10. Danielle Ofri, "Ashamed to Admit It," *Health Affairs* 29 (2010): 1549–51.

11. W. M. McDonnell and E. Guenther, "Narrative Review: Do State Laws Make It Easier to Say 'I'm Sorry'?" *Annals of Internal Medicine* 149 (2008): 811–16.

CHAPTER 6

1. Milt Freudenheim, "Adjusting, More M.D.'s Add M.B.A.," *New York Times*, September 6, 2011, http://www.nytimes.com/.

2. F. Davidoff, "Music Lessons: What Musicians Can Teach Doctors (and Other Health Professionals)," *Annals of Internal Medicine* 154 (2011): 426–29.

3. Physicians Foundation, "The Physicians' Perspective: Medical Practice (2008)," October 23, 2008, http://www.physiciansfoundation.org/.

4. "To Repeat: Doctors Could Hang It Up," editorial, *Investor's Business Daily*, March 17, 2010, http://www.investors.com/; "Physician Survey: Health Reform's Impact on Physician Supply and Quality of Medical Care," Medicus Firm Survey, 2010, http://www.themedicusfirm.com/.

5. W. H. Bylsma et al., "Where Have All the General Internists Gone?" *Journal of General Internal Medicine* 25 (2010): 1020–23.

6. D. Morra et al., "U.S. Physician Practices Versus Canadians: Spending Nearly Four Times As Much Money Interacting with Payers," *Health Affairs* 30 (2011): 1443–50.

7. L. P. Casalino, "What Does It Cost Physician Practices to Interact with Health Insurance Plans?" *Health Affairs* 28 (2009): w533–w543.

8. M. D. Tipping et al., "Where Did the Day Go?—A Time-Motion Study of Hospitalists," *Journal of Hospital Medicine* 5 (2010): 323–28.

9. Danielle Ofri, "When Computers Come Between Doctors and Patients," *Well* blog, New York Times.com, September 8, 2011, http://well.blogs.nytimes.com/.

10. J. Farber et al., "How Much Time Do Physicians Spend Providing Care Outside of Office Visits?" *Annals of Internal Medicine* 147 (2007): 693–98.

11. M. A. Chen et al., "Patient Care Outside of Office Visits: A Primary Care Physician Time Study," *Journal of General Internal Medicine* 26 (2011): 58–63.

12. "Women in Medicine" site, American Medical Association, http://www.ama-assn.org/.

13. "NRMP Historical Reports," National Residency Matching Program, http://www.nrmp.org/.

14. T. D. Shanafelt et al., "Burnout and Satisfaction with Work-Life Balance Among U.S. Physicians Relative to the General U.S. Population," *Archives of Internal Medicine* 172 (2012): 1–9.

15. M. R. Baldisseri, "Impaired Healthcare Professional," *Critical Care Medicine* 35 (2007): S106–16.

16. K. B. Gold and S. A. Teitelbaum, "Physicians Impaired by Substance Abuse Disorders," *Journal of Global Drug Policy and Practice* 2 (Summer 2008), http://www.globaldrugpolicy.org/.

17. S. D. Brown, M. J. Goske, and C. M. Johnson, "Beyond Substance Abuse: Stress, Burnout, and Depression as Causes of Physician Impairment and Disruptive Behavior," *Journal of the American College of Radiology* 6 (2009): 479–85.

18. C. P. West et al., "Association of Resident Fatigue and Distress with Perceived Medical Errors," *Journal of the American Medical Association* 302 (2009): 1294–1300; T. D. Shanafelt et al., "Burnout and Medical Errors Among American Surgeons," *Annals of Surgery* 251 (2010): 995–1000; T. D. Shanafelt et al., "Burnout and Self-Reported Patient Care in an Internal Medicine Residency Program," *Annals of Internal Medicine* 136 (2002): 358–67.

19. J. T. Prins et al., "Burnout, Engagement and Resident Physicians' Self-Reported Errors," *Psychology, Health, and Medicine* 14 (2009): 654–66.

20. M. R. DiMatteo et al., "Physicians' Characteristics Influence Patients' Adherence to Medical Treatment: Results from the Medical Outcomes Study," *Health Psychology* 12 (1993): 93–102.

21. D. Scheurer et al., "U.S. Physician Satisfaction: A Systematic Review," *Journal of Hospital Medicine* 9 (2009): 560–68; L. N. Dyrbye et al., "Work/Home Conflict and Burnout Among Academic Internal Medicine Physicians," *Archives of Internal Medicine* 171 (2011): 1207–9.

22. R. N. Remen, "Recapturing the Soul of Medicine," *Western Journal of Medicine* 174 (2001): 4–5.

23. C. M. Balch and T. Shanafelt, "Combating Stress and Burnout in Surgical Practice: A Review," *Advances in Surgery* 44 (2010): 29–47; T. D. Shanafelt, J. A. Sloan, and T. M. Habermann, "The Well-Being of Physicians," *American Journal of Medicine* 114 (2003): 513–19.

JULIA, PART SIX

1. John Stone, "Gaudeamus Igitur," *Journal of the American Medical Association* 249, no. 13 (1983): 1741–42.

CHAPTER 7

1. A. Kachalia and D. Studdert, "Professional Liability Issues in Graduate Medical Education," *Journal of the American Medical Association* 292 (2004): 1051–56.

2. R. A. Bailey, "Resident Liability in Medical Malpractice," *Annals of Emergency Medicine* 61, no. 1 (2013): 114–17.

3. C. K. Kane, "Medical Liability Claim Frequency: A 2007–2008 Snapshot of Physicians," AMA Policy Research Perspectives, www.ama-assn.org/.

4. A. B. Jena, "Malpractice Risk According to Physician Specialty," *New England Journal of Medicine* 365 (2011): 629–36.

5. R. B. Ferrell and T. R. Price, "Effects of Malpractice Suits on Physicians," in *Beyond Transference: When the Therapist's Real Life Intrudes*, Judith H. Gold and John C. Nemiah, eds. (Washington, DC: American Psychiatric Press, 1993), 141–58.

6. S. C. Charles, C. E. Pyskoty, and A. Nelson, "Physicians on Trial: Self-Reported Reactions to Malpractice Trials," *Western Journal of Medicine* 148 (1988): 358–60.

7. Sara C. Charles and Eugene Kennedy, *Defendant: A Psychiatrist on Trial for Medical Malpractice* (New York: Vintage Books, 1986), 7.

8. Ibid.

9. Charles, "Physicians on Trial"; S. C. Charles, "Sued and Nonsued Physicians' Self-Reported Reactions to Malpractice Litigation," *American Journal of Psychiatry* 142 (1985): 437–40.

10. S. C. Charles, "The Doctor-Patient Relationship and Medical Malpractice Litigation," *Bulletin of the Menninger Clinic* 57 (1993): 195–207.

11. S. C. Charles, "Malpractice Suits: Their Effect on Doctors, Patients, and Families," *Journal of the Medical Association of Georgia* 76 (1987): 171–72.

12. D. J. Brenner et al., "Computed Tomography—An Increasing Source of Radiation Exposure," *New England Journal of Medicine* 357 (2007): 2277–84.

13. Gilbert Welch et al., *Overdiagnosed: Making People Sick in the Pursuit of Health* (Boston: Beacon Press, 2011).

14. M. M. Mello et al., "National Costs of the Medical Liability System," *Health Affairs* 29 (2010): 1569–77.

15. M. K. Sethi et al., "The Prevalence and Costs of Defensive Medicine Among Orthopaedic Surgeons: A National Survey Study," *American Journal of Orthopaedics* 41 (2012): 69–73.

16. C. M. Balch et al., "Personal Consequences of Malpractice Lawsuits on American Surgeons," *Journal of the American College of Surgeons* 213 (2011): 657–67.

17. Charles and Kennedy, *Defendant*, 212.

18. Jena, "Malpractice Risk."

19. C. K. Cassel and S. H. Jain, "Assessing Individual Physician Performance: Does Measurement Suppress Motivation?" *Journal of the American Medical Association* 307 (2012): 2595–96.

20. Daniel H. Pink, *Drive: The Surprising Truth About What Motivates Us* (New York: Riverhead Books, 2011).

21. Danielle Ofri, "Quality Measures and the Individual Physician," *New England Journal of Medicine* 363 (2010): 606–7; Danielle Ofri, "Finding a Quality Doctor," *New York Times*, August 18, 2011.

22. A. Mostaghimi et al., "The Availability and Nature of Physician Information on the Internet," *Journal of General Internal Medicine* 25 (2010): 1152–56.

23. Danielle Ofri, *Singular Intimacies: Becoming a Doctor at Bellevue* (Boston: Beacon Press, 2009), 236.

JULIA, PART SEVEN

1. John Stone, "Gaudeamus Igitur," *Journal of the American Medical Association* 249, no. 13 (1983): 1741–42.

AFTERWORD

1. From Hippocrates, "Precepts," chapter 1, *Ancient Medicine. Airs, Waters, Places. Epidemics I & III. The Oath. Precepts. Nutriment.* W. H. S. Jones, trans. (Cambridge, MA: Harvard University Press, 1923).

2. Paul Oglesby, *The Caring Physician: The Life of Dr. Francis W. Peabody* (Boston: Francis A. Countway Library of Medicine, 1991).

Index

abandonment, 13
addiction, 10, 18–22, 113–19, 145–49, 159, 167–68
advance directives, 180–81
"Aequanimitas" (Osler), 4, 56, 212. See also *equanimitas*
AIDS. *See* HIV
alcoholism, 145–49, 167–69. *See also* addiction
alcohol (ETOH) withdrawal, 19
Alvarez, Maríssima (patient with excessive complaints), 16–18, 86
Amparo-Alvarado, Julia (heart-transplant patient), 23–28, 60–63, 95–97, 122–23, 140–42, 170–72, 202–9, 211
amygdala, 67–68, 74–75
anchoring bias, 2
anger: and communication, 14, 56; and empathy, 14–15, 18, 103–5, 147–48; and hospital slang, 18; patient-care consequences of, 147–50, 159, 210; and stress, 146–48. *See also* grief
Angie's List, 196
anticipatory grief, 123
Apert syndrome, 110
apology, 128, 133, 139. See also *On Apology*; shame
attribution bias, 2, 86–89

Becker, Ernest, 68, 75–76, 92–93
bedside manner, 52–56, 198
Bellevue Hospital Center: attending physicians, 53; author's residency at, 124; garden, 23; HIV/AIDS ward of, 45, 47; patient care commitment of, 140–42, 172; patient population of, 12, 15, 19, 140; psychiatric emergency room of, 40–43; rape-crisis program of, 6; time management at, 162; view of, as public hospital, 76

bias, 2, 13–15, 29–30, 86–89
blood clot. *See* pulmonary embolism
borderline personality disorder, 187–88, 192
boredom, 146–47, 150–51, 153
breast cancer, 179–85
burnout, 104–6, 148, 156–60, 163–64, 167, 169. *See also* grief; stress

cardiac arrest. *See* code
career shifting, 167–69
Carello, John (patient with drug addiction), 19–22
cello. *See* music
Charles, Sara (psychiatrist who was sued), 187–90, 192
CHF (congestive heart failure), 24–25, 60; treatment of, 95
Climer, Curtis (medical resident who was overwhelmed), 69–74, 143–44
clinical algorithms, 3, 131–32
clinical competency, 1
clinical curiosity, 53–54
clinical training. *See* medical education
code, 64–67, 117, 176; pediatric, 103–4
communication, 14, 26–27, 56, 137, 190
compassion, 4, 8–9, 10, 12. *See also* empathy
confidence, 13–14
congestive heart failure, 24–25, 60; treatment of, 95
continuing medical education (CME), 165–66, 168
cultural/ethnic identity, 16–18

Damasio, Antonio, 3
death: acceptance of, 102, 205–9; denial of, 26–28, 68, 75–76, 92–93, 119, 122–23; pervasiveness of, 107–8. *See also* grief
defensive medicine, 139, 178, 187, 190–92

denial, 61–62, 95, 122; of death, 26–28, 68, 75–76, 92–93, 119, 122–23
The Denial of Death (Becker), 68, 75–76, 92–93
detachment, 103–5, 107–8
diagnosis: accuracy improvements, 92; anchoring bias error in, 2; attribution bias in, 2, 86–89; difficulty telling, 25–28, 61–62, 127; incorrect, 85, 90–91, 175–77
disillusionment: and career shifting, 154, 167–69; and frustration, 146–47, 150–51; and health-care reform concerns, 153–54; and lack of stimulation, 152–53; and litigation, 192; and loss of empathy, 147–50, 159; and medical error, 160; and medical specialties, 154–57; and paperwork, 155–56; reduction programs, 163–66; and substance abuse, 19, 148–49, 158–59; and time management, 153–57
dissociative reaction, 69–74
DKA (diabetic ketoacidosis), 124–27, 138–39
doctor-patient relationship, 4–5, 133, 178, 186, 192–93, 210–11
Down syndrome, 111–13
dusky foot, 90–91

Easton, James (patient with severe ulcers), 11–12, 57–59
education. *See* medical education
Edwards, Isaac (patient who died alone), 113–19
embitterment, 148–49, 187
emergency room, 124–27, 146–49; psychiatric, 40–43
emotion, 2–3, 7–9, 31–33, 119–21, 211–12. *See also* anger; grief
empathy: and anger, 14–15, 103–5; and compassion, 4, 8–9, 10, 12, 111–13; and cultural/ethnic identity, 16–18; defined, 57; and expediency, 31–36; and fatigue, 30, 34, 70, 148, 169; and fear, 37; loss of, 30–36, 47, 147–50, 159; and medical education's hidden curriculum, 33–36; and mixed messages, 31–33; modeling, 53–56; and patient health outcomes, 56–57, 110–13; and personal bias, 13–15; and "self-induced" illness, 10, 18–22, 113–19, 146; and sense of self, 48; and

short-sightedness, 57–59; studies of, 49–50, 56–57; teaching, 29–30, 50–52; testing and measurement of, 29–30, 47–49, 50, 57. *See also* humor
enrichment, personal, 150–52, 166
equanimitas, 147, 210
error. *See* medical error
ethnic/cultural identity, 16–18
ETOH-WD. *See* alcohol withdrawal
Eva (pediatrics intern with dying baby), 98–106, 108–13, 121
evidence-based medicine, 3
expediency, 31–36

failure, 64–69, 74, 76–85
fatigue, 30, 34, 70, 148, 169
fear: and denial, 92; and empathy, 37; of failure, 64–67, 68–69, 74, 76–85; of litigation threat, 133, 139, 173–75, 177–78, 181–85, 187; positive aspects of, 93–94; processing of, 67–68, 74–76; and vigilance, 93–94
Finding Meaning in Medicine groups, 165
Florida Hospital group, 163–66
frustration, 146–48, 150–51, 160–62, 200–201
full-disclosure policies, 127

gallows humor. *See* humor
"Gaudeamus Igitur" (Stone), 171, 209
grief: acknowledgment of, 108–9, 138–39, 200–201, 205–9; anticipatory, 123; and detachment, 103–5, 107–8; and embitterment, 148–49, 187; and emotional depletion, 119–21; gaining strength from, 200–201; and isolation, 102, 119; and medical care decisions, 98–105, 108–13, 122–23; and PTSD, 105–6; suppression of, 99–100, 102–5. *See also* anger; disillusionment
Groopman, Jerome, 2, 5, 85, 88, 210
Guatemala, 141, 200, 207
guilt: and denial, 26, 61–62; and medical error, 87–89; positive aspects of, 91–92; and shame, 125–29, 135–36, 138–39

Hamlin, Josephine (homeless woman who was raped), 7–9
Harvard Medical School, 50–52
health-care reform, 153–54
heart transplant. *See* organ transplant
hernia, inguinal, 114–17

Hickam's dictum, 88
Hippocrates, 211
Hippocratic oath, 7
HIV, 45–47, 146
The House of God (Shem), 43–45
How Doctors Think (Groopman), 2, 85, 88
How Patients Think (book series), 85
humanities studies, 49–50
humiliation. *See* shame
humor: and anger, 18; as emotional release, 39, 44–45; and inclusion, 37–38, 43; as shield, 16, 37, 40–43, 45–47; as teaching tool, 37–40, 43
hyperkalemia, 64–67

ICU (intensive care unit): congestive heart failure patient in, 62, 95, 205–9; hyperkalemia patient in, 64–67; misdiagnosed patient in, 176, 200–201; patient population of, 174; pediatric, 103–5
integrated clerkships, 50–52
Internet, 2, 196–99
Intern Game, 34
isolation, 102, 119

jargon, hospital, 36, 177
Jefferson Medical College Scale of Empathy (JSE), 48–49, 50, 57
Joanne (ER doctor who developed alcoholism), 143–49, 167–69
joy, 121, 142, 170–72, 179, 210–11

Landon, Cynthia (patient who wanted weight-loss pills), 13–15
Lazare, Aaron, 128, 133
litigation: and disillusionment, 192; and the doctor-patient relationship, 192–93, 210–11; emotional toll of, 185–91; fear of, 133, 139, 173–75, 177–78, 181–85, 187; financial burden of, 192; patient care consequences of, 139, 154–57, 178, 187, 190–92; rates of, 193; and risk aversion, 154–57, 192
love, 101–2, 120
Lyme disease, 175–76

Maimonides. *See* oath of Maimonides
malpractice suits. *See* litigation
manipulation, 13–14
Manning, Yvonne (patient who died of breast cancer, daughter filed suit), 178–85

MCAT (Medical College Admission Test), 52
medical education: and empathy loss, 30–36, 47, 147–50, 159; hidden curriculum of, 33–36; humanities studies, 49–50; integrated clerkships, 50–52; medical error education, 136–37; and medical terminology, 36–38; mixed messages of, 31–33; multiculturalism studies, 52–54; self-discipline demands of, 18; on shame, 136–37; and slang/gallows humor, 37–40, 43; structure of, 3–4, 32; and time management, 74–75, 143–45, 160–62
medical error: and disillusionment, 160; emotional toll of, 2, 124–27, 134–36, 175–76; and guilt, 87–89; medical education on, 136–37; reduction, 139; studies, 137–38
medical experience, 3
Medicine in Translation (Ofri), 26–27, 62–63, 97, 203, 206–7
Mercedes (patient who was thought to have Lyme disease), 175–76, 199–201
misdiagnosis, 85, 90–91, 175–77; anchoring bias error in, 2, 86–89; consequences of, 87–90, 124–27, 176–77; rates of, 92
Morbidity and Mortality (M&M) conferences, 54, 133–34, 193
multiculturalism studies, 52–54
music, 151–53

Natalie (psychiatric patient who attempted suicide), 187–89
negative emotions, 2

oath of Maimonides, 7, 10
Occam's razor, 88
Ofri, Danielle, 26–27, 62–63, 97, 200–201, 203, 206–7
On Apology (Lazare), 128, 133
oncologists, 107–9, 134–36, 183–84
online ratings, 196–99
organ transplant, 25–28, 62–63, 95, 142, 170–72, 202–5
Osler, William, 3–4, 56, 57, 147, 210, 212
Overdiagnosed (Welch), 191–92
overdose, drug, 19–22, 76–83
overwhelmed, feeling: and decision making, 74–75; and empathy loss, 159; and fatigue, 30, 34, 70, 148, 169; and

medical education structure, 32; and revulsion, 7–9, 10–12, 40–43, 57–58; and time pressures, 83–84

Paolini, Herdley (psychologist who created physician wellness program), 162–66
pain, perception of, 29–30
patient: emotion, 211–12; empathy and health outcomes of, 56–57, 110–13; patient-doctor relationship, 192–93, 210–11; patient-satisfaction surveys, 193, 196–99; personality traits, 12–15; view of misdiagnosis, 85
patient care consequences: and anger, 37, 132–33, 147–50, 159, 210; of grief, 98–105, 108–13, 122–23; of litigation, 139, 154–57, 178, 187, 190–92; of shame, 132–33
Peabody, Francis, 212
peaked T waves, 66–67
personal bias, 13–15
personal enrichment, 150–52
personality traits: patient, 12–15; physician, 133
physician evaluations, 196–99
Physicians Foundation study, 153–54
positive emotions, 2, 210–11
posttraumatic stress disorder (PTSD), 105–6, 108
Potter syndrome, 99, 101
pride, 124–25, 175–76
prognosis, difficulty telling, 25–28, 61–62, 127
pulmonary embolism, 86–89, 91–92

quality-measures movement, 3, 193–95

racial bias, 29–30
Rand Corporation study, 160
rape, 6–9, 141
Remen, Rachael Naomi, 165
report cards, 193–95
respect, 53–56
revulsion, 7–9, 10–12, 40–43, 57–58
risk management, 173–75, 181–85. See also litigation
Robert Wood Johnson Medical School Humanism and Professionalism study, 49–50

sadness. See grief
"self-induced" illness, 10, 18–22, 113–19, 146
self-judgment, 199–201
shame: and apology, 128, 133, 139; averting, 139; benefits of, 132, 139; and expectations, 130–31; and guilt, 125–29, 135–36, 138–39; medical education on, 136–37; patient care consequences of, 132–33
Shem, Samuel, 43–44
short-sightedness, 57–59
Singular Intimacies (Ofri), 200–201
slang/gallows humor. See humor
sleep, lack of, 30, 34, 70, 148, 169
Spencer, Frank, 54–56
Starling curve, 23–24
stereotypes and stereotyping, 3–4, 89–90
Stone, John, 171, 209
stress, 69–74, 102–5, 146–48, 164–65
stress management programs, 75, 165–67
suicide attempt, 76–83, 187–89

time management: and disillusionment, 153–57; and feeling overwhelmed, 83–84, 160–62; and medical school education, 74–75, 143–45, 161–62; and productivity goals, 89

University of California at San Francisco School of Medicine, 50
University of Minnesota Medical School, 51
University of Rochester, 108–9

weight-loss pills, 13–15
Welch, Gilbert, 191–92
wellness programs, 163–66
"What Musicians Teach Doctors" (Annals of Internal Medicine), 152–53
Wilton, Beverly (patient with missed pulmonary embolism), 86, 87–88, 90, 91–92
Winicott, Donald, 129
worried-well, 13–15, 86–88

Zhong, Hao (patient who attempted suicide and was transferred to Mount Sinai), 76–83